AF252138

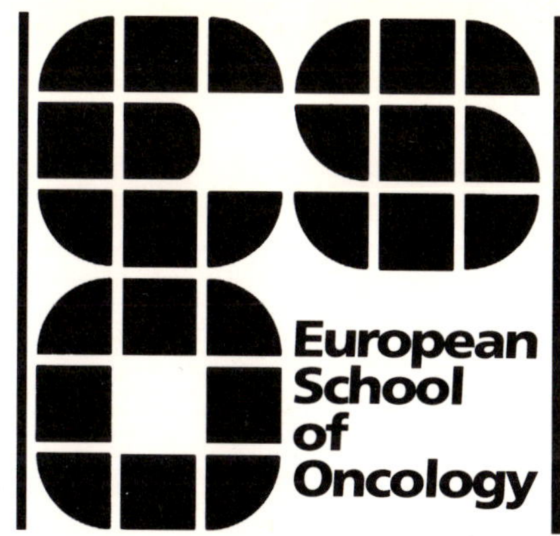

Monographs

Series Editor: U. Veronesi

The European School of Oncology gratefully acknowledges sponsorship for the Task Force received from STERLING WINTHROP

P. Workman (Ed.)

New Approaches in Cancer Pharmacology: Drug Design and Development, Vol. II

With 33 Figures and 10 Tables

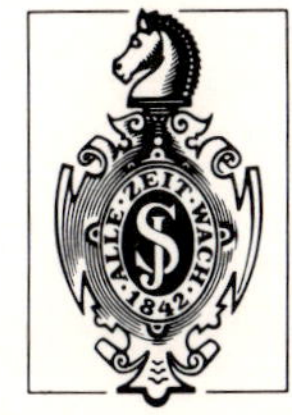

Springer-Verlag
Berlin   Heidelberg   New York
London   Paris   Tokyo
Hong Kong   Barcelona
Budapest

Professor Paul Workman (Chairman and Editor)*

Cancer Research Campaign Beatson Laboratories
CRC Department of Medical Oncology
University of Glasgow
Alexander Stone Building
Garscube Estate, Switchback Road
Bearsden, Glasgow G61 1BD, UK

Dr. Maurizio D'Incalci (Co-chairman)

Istituto Mario Negri
Via Eritrea 62
20157 Milano, Italy

*current address: ZENECA Pharmaceuticals, Cancer Research Department,
 Mereside, Alderley Park, Macclesfield, Cheshire SK10 4TG, UK

ISBN 3-540-58153-7 Springer-Verlag Berlin Heidelberg New York
ISBN 0-387-58153-7 Springer-Verlag New York Berlin Heidelberg

Library of Congress Cataloging-in-Publication Data
New approaches in cancer pharmacology: drug design and development, Vol. II / P. Workman (ed.)
    (Monographs / European School of Oncology)
Includes bibliographical references.
    ISBN 3-540-58153-7 (alk. paper)
    ISBN 0-387-58153-7 (alk. paper)
1. Antineoplastic agents--Design. I. Workman, P. (Paul) II. Series: Monographs (European School of Oncology) [DNLM:
1. Antineoplastic Agents--pharmacology. 2. Drug Design. QV 269 N53167 1994] RC271.C5N43 1994 616.99'4061--dc20
DNLM/DLC for Library of Congress

Typesetting: Camera ready by editor
Printing: Druckhaus Beltz, Hemsbach/Bergstraße; Binding: J. Schäffer GmbH & Co. KG, Grünstadt
SPIN: 10091134   19/3130 - 5 4 3 2 1 0 — Printed on acid-free paper

Foreword

The European School of Oncology came into existence to respond to a need for information, education and training in the field of the diagnosis and treatment of cancer. There are two main reasons why such an initiative was considered necessary. Firstly, the teaching of oncology requires a rigorously multidisciplinary approach which is difficult for the Universities to put into practice since their system is mainly disciplinary orientated. Secondly, the rate of technological development that impinges on the diagnosis and treatment of cancer has been so rapid that it is not an easy task for medical faculties to adapt their curricula flexibly.

With its residential courses for organ pathologies and the seminars on new techniques (laser, monoclonal antibodies, imaging techniques etc.) or on the principal therapeutic controversies (conservative or mutilating surgery, primary or adjuvant chemotherapy, radiotherapy alone or integrated), it is the ambition of the European School of Oncology to fill a cultural and scientific gap and, thereby, create a bridge between the University and Industry and between these two and daily medical practice.

One of the more recent initiatives of ESO has been the institution of permanent study groups, also called task forces, where a limited number of leading experts are invited to meet once a year with the aim of defining the state of the art and possibly reaching a consensus on future developments in specific fields of oncology.

The ESO Monograph series was designed with the specific purpose of disseminating the results of these study group meetings, and providing concise and updated reviews of the topic discussed.

It was decided to keep the layout relatively simple, in order to restrict the costs and make the monographs available in the shortest possible time, thus overcoming a common problem in medical literature: that of the material being outdated even before publication.

Umberto Veronesi
Chairman Scientific Committee
European School of Oncology

Dedication

This volume is dedicated to two of our fellow soldiers in the war against cancer who were themselves lost to the disease in 1993: the French medical oncologist Michel Clavel, who was an active early clinical trialist and a great supporter of cancer pharmacology, and the American pharmaceutical company scientist Gerald Grindey, who was an insightful advocate of experimental chemotherapy and rational drug development.
The editor also acknowledges the influence of two others who departed in 1993: the clinician, biologist and philosopher Lewis Thomas and the musician Frank Zappa.

Contents

Introduction

Paul Workman

Cancer Research Campaign Department of Medical Oncology, University of Glasgow, CRC Beatson Laboratories, Garscube Estate, Switchback Road, Bearsden, Glasgow G61 1BD, United Kingdom

In my introduction to the preceding volume published in 1992 [1], I referred to the exhilarating pace at which our understanding of the molecular basis of cancer is advancing and the marvellous opportunity this presents us with - to exploit such knowledge in the rational development of totally novel therapies which should have enhanced efficacy and selectivity against the major solid tumours. At the same time, the deployment of sound pharmacological principles, often innervated by modern molecular biology techniques, continues to offer valuable improvements to the design and optimal utilisation of the conventionally acting cancer drugs which remain the mainstay of current cancer chemotherapy.

The previous monograph covered DNA sequene and gene-specific drugs (M. D'Incalci et al.), antisense and antigene oligonucleotides targeted to oncogenes (C. Hélène), prospects for biological and gene therapies (K. Sikora and A. Guiterrez), membrane and signal transduction targets (J.A. Hickman), design of novel anti-endocrine agents (M. Jarman), design of novel bioreductive drugs (P. Workman), therapeutic drug monitoring and dose optimisation in oncology (M.J. Egorin), and current strategies in anticancer drug discovery within the EORTC (G. Schwartsmann). Continuing with our brief of examining progress and predicting future trends in cancer pharmacology generally, and in drug design and development in particular, we have selected a wide range of exciting new topics for the present volume.

The opening chapter by Maurizio D'Incalci (Milano) covers selective aspects of the pharmacological evaluation of new anticancer agents. The emphasis here is on the importance of choosing the most relevant model systems, particularly as we begin to develop drugs acting on novel molecular targets. The move is generally towards mechanism-based drug hunting strategies with critical input of molecular biology expertise. Screening cascades must be established which can take in large synthetic chemical or natural product collections, recently extended by combinatorial peptide, oligonucleotide and oligosaccharide libraries, and then rapidly reduce these enormous numbers of compounds to a more manageable quantity for detailed study. These screens must be configured in such a way as to pick out weak hits acting on the selected molecular target, and after this to progressively refine the hits into more potent and biochemically selective leads displaying the desired activity against intact cells. Finally, the appropriate therapeutic effect must be detected by *in vivo* screens which at the same time challenge the ability of the drug candidate to run the gauntlet of pharmacokinetics and normal tissue toxicity. At the front end of such cascades pharmaceutical companies frequently operate at throughputs of several thousand compounds per week. In addition to high throughput screening, the development of structure-based approaches at an early stage of drug discovery programmes is increasingly common, involving X-ray cyrstallography and nuclear magnetic resonance spectroscopy techniques. D'Incalci stresses the importance of selecting cell culture and whole animal models which are in tune with the relevant mechanims. For example, the growth of a cell line or *in vivo* tumour should be driven by the target oncogene or growth factor. This may necessitate molecular characterization of existing tumour models or even creation of new ones by genetic engineering. The use of human tumour xenografts in immunosuppressed mice continues to be important for *in vivo* testing. Amid concerns about the retention of critical functional properties by tissue culture-derived lines, further work is required to develop more sophisticated and biologically relevant models which are nevertheless suitable for routine drug evaluation.

The classical DNA-interactive drugs are essentially non-selective in their molecular action and fail to discriminate between tumour and normal DNA. Any selective antitumour effects are dependent on events downstream of DNA binding, particularly the way in which the cell recognises and then processes the damage. Thus existing DNA-damaging drugs are largely "information-neutral". Here, Stephen Neidle (Sutton) lays out the potential for "information-reading" DNA-binding drugs which might for example recognise unique base sequences in DNA that have arisen by point mutation or translocation. His contribution updates and extends those of D'Incalci and Hélène in the earlier book, with particular emphasis on structural aspects. Anti-sense RNA, triple-helix DNA-forming oligonucleotides and sequence-specific natural product approaches are compared. The challenge is emphasised by the calculation that in order to achieve total specificity against a chosen genetic sequence, it is necessary to recognise 15-18 contiguous base pairs.

Of the currently used "information-neutral" DNA-binding drugs, cisplatin is one of the most effective. Nevertheless, further refinement of the drug molecule can be valuable, as exemplified by carboplatin in which the kidney toxicity is absent. In his review of the discovery of improved platinum drugs, Ken Harrap (Sutton) focuses in particular on progress and challenges in the design of platinum drugs with oral activity and with the ability to circumvent both intrinsic and acquired drug resistance. Success in these areas at the preclinical level is due in part to the judicious selection of appropriate models. He suggests that further advances may involve exploitation of molecular biological aspects of resistance.

Taking a somewhat different though related personal perspective from the review by John Hickman in the previous monograph, the following chapter by Garth Powis (Tucson) analyses the promise and problems of inhibitors of signal transduction for cancer treatment. He points out that not only is it possible to identify drugs which might block oncoprotein function, one can also take the approach of inhibiting signalling pathways that are activated downstream of the oncogene product. For example, inhibitors of oncogene and growth factor-stimulated phospholipases are cited as examples of such "surrogate" downstream targets. Degeneracy of signal transduction pathways in normal cells may protect them from side-effects, as exemplified by recent transgenic mice studies in which proto-oncogenes were knocked out without lethal effect. A cytostatic rather than cytotoxic effect of signalling inhibitors may be envisaged, but cell death could ensue in certain circumstances. Similarly, although the presence of multiple genetic changes within individual human cancers suggests that more than one anti-signalling drug would be needed to suppress growth, in fact gene transfer studies suggest that correction of a single defect may be sufficient. However, development of resistance to the new signal transduction drugs is quite possible, especially given the genetic instability of cancer cells and the potential for the induction of alternative signalling pathways.

Many oncogene products and growth factor receptors contain tyrosine kinase domains which are essential for biological activity. This is consistent with the increased level of tyrosine phosphorylation commonly observed in tumour cells. Moreover, in some human cancers the levels of certain tyrosine kinases, such as those associated with epidermal growth factor receptor and erbB2, are independent prognostic variables, suggesting a direct link to tumour growth. It is not surprising therefore that the discovery and development of tyrosine kinase inhibitors is being hotly pursued by both pharmaceutical companies and academic groups. Paul Workman and colleagues (Glasgow) illustrate how considerable progress has been made by combining high throughput screening and structure-based strategies and by the use of molecular biology to create recombinant proteins and transfected cell lines. Various interesting chemical structures have been identified as tyrosine kinase inhibitors. These include the tyrphostin type compounds which illustrate that considerable specificity can be achieved across different kinases. *In vivo* antitumour activity has been seen with certain inhibitors and clinical trials are anticipated shortly. Meanwhile dramatic progress has been made in our understanding of the precise mechanism by which receptor tyrosine kinases (and also the src oncoprotein) are able to signal to the nucleus. This involves interaction of the src homology domain (SH2) of the adaptor protein grb with a highly specific phosphotyrosine residue in the ligand-activated, autophosphorylated growth factor receptor. Information then flows via a series of protein-protein interactions and phosphorylation events from grb → sos → ras → raf → MEK → MAP kinase → transcription factors → gene expression. This knowledge yields up yet more targets for drug discovery. Mutant ras was already known to be an important locus and very promising recent results show that peptide mimetics can inhibit the farnesylation reaction, which is essential for ras function, within intact cells. Moreover, specificity is seen for cells with mutant versus normal *ras* genes. In seeking to define the most optimal point in the above-mentioned pathway for therapeutic intervention, our assessment of the likely therapeutic cost-benefit ratio is made difficult by the branched nature or "cross-talk" displayed. Although molecular genetics can help greatly in the choice of targets for optimal selectivity, in the final analysis only experience with real drug candidates in our hands will answer this vital question.

"In the midst of life we are in death." This fundamental truth of general biology is equally apposite for malignant cells. The growth rate of both normal and tumour tissues is governed by the balance of cell proliferation, differentiation and death. Kerr, Wyllie and Currie published their now classic paper on programmed cell death or apoptosis in 1972, but it is only in the last couple of years that the true significance for cancer research and treatment has been fully grasped. Of particular significance is the discovery at the molecular level that oncogenes, tumour suppressor genes and growth factors regulate death as well as division. Oncogenes such as *myc*, *bcl2* and *abl* and suppressor genes such as *p53* are intimately involved in a finely tuned fashion. Wilfried Bursch (Vienna) reviews the link between cell suicide and cancer therapy, both current and future, in his chapter. The ability of cells to engage the apoptotic pathway is a crucial factor in the efficacy and normal tissue toxicity of existing cancer drugs. Response to DNA damaging agents is strongly influenced by the *p53* gene product which acts as a transcription factor regulating genome fidelity at the G1-S cell cycle checkpoint. Very recent data show that wild type p53 protein turns on expression of the *waf/cip* gene, the product of which binds to and inhibits cyclin-dependent kinases which phosphorylate key cell cycle control proteins, such as the retinoblastoma gene product Rb. As we continue to unravel the signalling pathways involved in apoptosis, it seems inevitable that this information will help us not only to understand but also to modulate responsiveness of tumours and normal tissues to cytotoxic agents. In addition, a molecular description of programmed cell death will undoubtedly generate novel targets for innovative drug discovery programmes in cancer and other diseases.

The old concept of a "magic bullet" uniquely specific for cancer cells is most often discussed in the context of antibody therapy. Reviewing this topic in the final chapter, Robert Hawkins (Cambridge) points out that the clinical use of antibodies for targeted cancer therapy has achieved some success but has also revealed several problems. These latter include the immunogenicity of rodent antibodies, poor tumour penetration by macromolecules and the lack of entirely specific tumour antigens. Recombinant DNA techniques are now revolutionising the design of therapeutic antibodies. Humanisation is used to eliminate immunogenicity and miniaturisation to improve uptake. Recently, phage display technology has been used for rapid and direct production of antibodies. Selection of antibodies with properties such as high affinity or slow off-rate can be achieved with this technology. Advances in protein engineering have improved production, for example in bacteria. Fusion proteins consisting of antibodies linked to novel effector functions can also be manufactured by this means. The twin problems of penetration and antigenic heterogeneity may be simultaneously overcome by antibody-directed enzyme prodrug therapy (ADEPT), in which an antibody-enzyme conjugate targets the tumour and an inert prodrug is then activated selectively at the tumour site. Bispecific antibodies which recruit natural effectors and immunotoxins continue to be of interest. Antibodies may also be used to target therapeutic genes and appropriate vectors can be employed for the production of antibody-based molecules *in vivo*.

It is frustrating that there is a significant delay between any breakthrough in basic science and the exploitation of that knowledge in medical treatment. Although the delay is certainly shortening, the route from a newly cloned cancer gene to a designer cancer drug is a long and tortuous one. However, as the human genome is due to be mapped by the year 2000 and advances in molecular oncology and reverse genetics continue to provide new targets for innovative therapy, we can have considerable grounds for optimism that we should be looking forward to many exciting new ideas undergoing clinical evaluation in the coming decade.

Acknowledgements

I am grateful to my Task Force members for their time and enthusiastic commitment to this project. On their behalf I would like to acknowledge the staff of the European School of Oncology for their help, especially Vlatka Majstorovic for highly efficient organisation and Marije de Jager for painstaking and patient editorial support. Margaret Jenkins in my office in Glasgow provided invaluable coordination skills. The city of Venice was once again the perfect backdrop and catalyst for our deliberations. Finally, I am pleased to acknowledge Sterling Winthrop for their generous support of the Task Force.

REFERENCE

1   Workman P (ed) New Approaches in Cancer Pharmacology: Drug Design and Development. European School of Oncology Monograph Series, Springer-Verlag, Berlin 1992

Experimental Models to Investigate Novel Anticancer Drugs

Maurizio D'Incalci

Chairman of the Pharmacology and Molecular Mechanisms Group (PAMM) of the EORTC, Istituto di Ricerche Farmacologiche "Mario Negri", Via Eritrea 62, 20157 Milan, Italy

In the last decade our knowledge of tumour biology has increased dramatically. The development of molecular genetic techniques has made possible the identification of key proteins playing a role in the regulation of proliferation and differentiation, and in some cases the cellular pathways responsible for neoplastic transformation have been elucidated. This new scientific knowledge is becoming exploitable for the design of novel drugs, acting as specific inhibitors of these pathways. Various approaches to rational design are discussed elsewhere in this volume and in the previous monograph.

It should be remarked, however, that the design of new anticancer agents is still at an early stage. It is therefore still impossible to entirely replace the random screening system with rational drug design. Nevertheless, the identification of some new targets has made it possible to start using biochemical assays to identify potential novel drugs. For example, the recent evidence that DNA-topoisomerase enzymes are the targets of many active antineoplastic drugs, has prompted the development of biochemical assays to identify new inhibitors of these enzymes. The same approach is currently pursued for other enzymes (e.g. enzymes of signal transduction pathways) or growth factor receptors [1] and it is conceivable that by combining the ingenuity of medicinal chemistry with more modern drug design methods - based on knowledge of three-dimensional structures of the macromolecules - more potent and specific inhibitors will be obtained.

The identification of many compounds specifically active on relevant molecular targets, which play a role in neoplastic growth and differentiation, is in progress. But it is wise to anticipate that the majority of these will be extremely toxic as most of these targets play an important role also in many physiological processes occurring in normal cells.

If new compounds are selected because of their ability to inhibit a specific target molecule, it will be important in addition to develop cellular and *in vivo* tumour models which are suitable for adequate testing. If, for example, a new compound is selected because of its ability to bind a specific receptor, thus inhibiting the function of a ligand implicated in the neoplastic growth, it will be necessary to test this compound against *in vitro* tumour cell lines or *in vivo* mouse tumours or xenografts which exhibit that particular receptor. It appears therefore that while new mechanistically different anticancer agents are being developed, there should be a parallel development of *ad hoc* preclinical systems for *in vitro* and *in vivo* testing.

In this chapter the preclinical *in vitro* and *in vivo* systems which have been used in the past or which are currently used will be discussed, providing some examples of potentially useful new experimental models for testing drugs designed to hit a specific crucial target.

In Vitro Systems

A range of murine and human cell lines have been used for many years to identify and investigate new potential cytotoxic and cytostatic agents.

Some mouse leukaemia cell lines such as P388 and L1210 have been employed extensively because of their rapid growth rate and also be

1975 -1985

1985 up to now

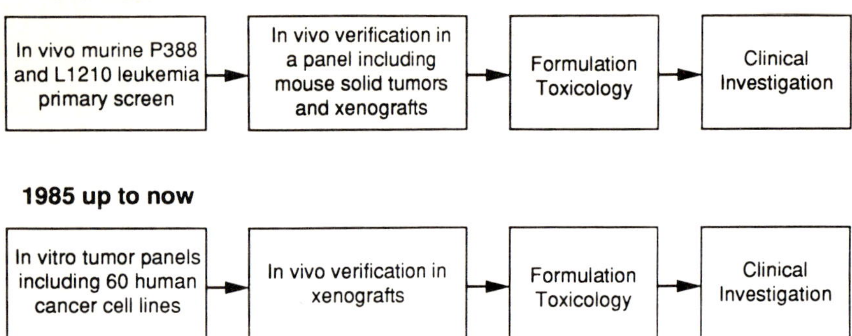

Fig. 1. Preclinical drug development strategies used by the NCI from 1975 to 1985 and from 1985 up till now

cause they could be reliably transplanted in mice, thus enabling the routine *in vivo* testing of compounds possessing antiproliferative properties.

Due to the relatively low number of anticancer agents with human solid tumour activity identified by the screening programme based on these murine leukaemia cell lines, in 1985 the US NCI activated a new screening programme based on the use of human cancer cell lines (Fig. 1) [2-4]. The change was prompted by the observation that most of the available clinically effective anticancer drugs are active mainly against leukaemia or lymphoma and not against the majority of solid human tumours. This could be perhaps due to the fact that the initial selection of drugs was done on the basis of the activity against a murine leukaemia. The possibility of using other solid rodent tumours growing *in vitro* and *in vivo* appeared a possible alternative, but it was still questionable whether a limited number of individual mouse tumours could adequately mimic the sensitivity of human neoplasms. The use of a large number of solid mouse tumours and of solid human tumours transplanted in nude mice was only a theoretical alternative, since the cost of a random screening on such animal models would have been prohibitive, considering the high number of compounds that are to be tested. Random screening is, in fact, a rather inefficient method to identify a new anticancer agent and it is unlikely that success can be achieved by testing a low number of compounds.

These considerations led the Division of Cancer Treatment of the NCI to set up the currently ongoing disease-oriented primary screening programme with the use of a large number of cell lines derived from human malignant tumours. Having evaluated several methods to assess the antiproliferative activity of a

compound after 48 h incubation, they selected the protein assay endpoint using sulforhodamine B staining. The assay was validated using 175 known compounds which were also employed to determine the reproducibility of the assays over time. The methods were automated in order to screen a very large number of compounds and data analysis was focussed on the goal of identifying selective cytototoxicity against particular tumour types [2-4]. The 60 cell lines are representative of all the major human cancer types with the exception of breast, prostate adenocarcinoma and squamous cell carcinoma. A further increase in the number of cell lines can be implemented in future to cover these additional important human tumours.

Although it is still too early to evaluate the success of the new screening initiative, as some compounds have been selected for further *in vivo* evaluation only recently, the screening procedure has been found to be feasible and has also generated some scientifically interesting observations. One of the most interesting findings is related to the pattern of activity of different compounds according to their mode of action. Weinstein et al. [5] designed a neural network capable of predicting a drug's mode of action from its pattern of activity across the range of cell lines. Six categories of mechanism of action were selected (i.e., alkylating agents, topoisomerase I inhibitors, topoisomerase II inhibitors, RNA/DNA antimetabolites, DNA antimetabolites and antimitotic agents) and a seventh category represented an unknown mechanism of action different from those listed above. The data base was formulated from a list of drugs whose putative mode of action was described in the scientific literature. The network predicted the categories of 129 out of 141 agents correctly (91.5%). This success is very high considering that in some cases the mode of action is not unequivocally established and it is impossible to ensure that the assignment to a given category is valid to the same extent in all cell lines. The impressive statistical significance of the prediction opens the possibility that once a novel compound is selected, the comparison of the pattern of activity in different cell lines with that in the data base can provide an indication of the mode of action of the new agent. It will be particularly interesting to discover whether the pattern of sensitivity reflects specific aspects of the biology of the cell lines. For instance it may be that the expression of certain oncogenes confers sensitivity to some drugs but not to others. Studies are in progress at the NCI to characterise the 60 human cell lines from a biological and biochemical point of view and then it might be possible to attempt to correlate the pattern of drug sensitivity to peculiar biological features of the human tumour cell lines.

Although the large panel of the cancer cell lines is theoretically representative of the various human neoplasms, a note of caution is suggested by the consideration that the established cell lines may have lost some of the relevant biological properties and drug sensitivity features of the human tumours they derive from. It is in fact known that established cell lines represent a selection of tumour cells which have adapted to the in vitro conditions and do not necessarily represent the total cancer cell populations present in the original human tumour. In addition, because of the genetic instability of tumour cells, mutations can easily occur, thereby modifying the biological and biochemical properties of the cell lines.

Another interesting system is that of primary cultures which probably mimic better the characteristics of the tumour they derive from and therefore are very useful to investigate specific biological and pharmacological research endpoints [see for example ref. 6]. However, they cannot be realistically employed for drug screening as they require very specialised and sophisticated techniques, difficult to apply on a large scale. In addition, in most cases only small tumour biopsies are available and thus only a limited number of compounds could be tested.

A possible general drawback of the use of cultured cancer cells to test new drugs is that some drugs would score as inactive because they require metabolic activation not occurring in cells grown in vitro. The cytotoxicity of some drugs can be different in vitro and in vivo because of differences in the concentrations of substrates which may enhance or antagonise the drug effects. For example the levels of folic acid in regular tissue culture growth medium are approximately 100 times those present in human plasma, thus possibly modifying the efficacy of antifolates.

There is an increasing body of experimental evidence suggesting that the behaviour of cancer cells is different if they are attached to plastic or to biological substrates such as collagen IV or fibronectin and even more so if they are cocultured with normal cells. Therefore a limitation of an in vitro cytotoxicity assay, performed by exposing cancer cell lines growing in the usual way in plastic petri dishes, is that if a drug works by modifying the interaction between the neoplastic cell and components of extracellular matrix [7,8] or by interfering with the communication between the cancer and the normal cells, a compound may appear inactive, but only because of the inadequacy of the test system. This may also apply to many compounds that act on the immune system or interfere with endothelial cell functions.

Although all these potential limitations of the in vitro screening procedures which are currently used are recognised by the majority of scientists working in the field, it should be accepted that a screening system in which many thousands of compounds are tested must necessarily be simple, quick and inexpensive. Therefore from a pragmatic point of view the NCI screening programme, particularly if a better characterisation of the cell lines is carried out (i.e., identification of oncogene expression and biochemical determinants of drug sensitivity and resistance), has considerable value and will hopefully facilitate the discovery of novel drugs. It should also be pointed out that the in vitro screening system is the only one which can be realistically used to identify the activity of extracts of natural products. In fact in most cases very small amounts of the active principle are present in the extracts and it is essential to be able to detect any activity in vitro in order to purify and identify the active component. The mode of action of potential cytotoxic and antiproliferative compounds extracted from natural sources is generally unknown and is often discovered several years after the identification of the active principle. It is therefore difficult to conceive of identifying these compounds with methods other than *in vitro* cytotoxicity assays. For other compounds it may instead be possible to integrate a random screening approach with other methods specifically designed to identify compounds acting against a given target.

With specific classes of compounds it may be useful to use *in vitro* growing cells which are genetically manipulated in a desired fashion. For example, it may be appropriate to use cells overexpressing a specific receptor, or a particular protein which is the supposed molecular target of drug action. It may also be of interest to use cells which have a deficient or no expression of enzymes involved in the protection of the cells (e.g. a DNA repair enzyme) or overexpression of enzymes which activate and enhance drug cytotoxicity [9,10].

By using oncogene transformed cells it may be possible to investigate specific inhibitors of signalling pathways mediated by growth factors and oncogene products. For example herbimycin B was recently found to be able to selectively inhibit the growth of *src* or *abl* transformed cells in serum-free medium [11].

Genetically manipulated cells can be extremely useful tools to identify new drugs acting by a specific mechanism but they are not necessarily representative of the complex tumour biology of human tumours. Therefore compounds found to be active against one of these cell lines should be tested also in other *in vitro* and *in vivo* experimental models before clinical development.

In Vivo Systems

We have already indicated some of the drawbacks in the use of mouse leukaemias for the primary screening of new anticancer agents. The high sensitivity of P388 and L1210 leukaemias to antiproliferative agents is likely to be related to the rapid growth rate of these tumours. The more general issue of to what extent murine tumours are representative of human tumours, which was in part discussed in the previous section, is still open to debate [12]. No demonstration exists that the lack of success in identifying effective new anticancer agents for human solid cancers is due to the use of murine tumours for primary screening. The primary screening was done using murine leukaemias and it is a matter of fact that several effective agents are available with proven activity against human leukaemias. The use of solid mouse tumours for screening purposes has been limited and we do not know how well they predict the drug sensitivity of human tumours. However, some of the solid mouse tumours do show a pattern of drug sensitivity similar to that of some human solid tumours. Most of them are not very sensitive to anticancer agents and cannot be cured if chemotherapy is started when the tumours are clinically manifest [13].

It may be that human xenografts are more representative experimental models as their histopathological features are often very closely related to the human tumours they derive from [14]. However, as far as the sensitivity to drugs is concerned, it is still unknown if they are good predictors for human tumours. It is known that some biological features of the human tumours do change after transplantation to mice. For example, the metastatic potential of human xenografts is often very low even if the original tumour was highly metastatic in the patient. This may be related to the site of inoculation of the tumour. In fact, recent evidence suggests that the pattern of metastasis of orthotopically transplanted nude mice is more closely related to that occurring in humans than is the case for subcutaneously or intramuscularly transplanted tumours [15]. It may be worthwhile underlining also that the sensitivity to anticancer agents has been reported to be dependent upon the orthotopic and ectopic environment [16], suggesting that the results obtained by testing compounds against subcutaneously transplanted human tumours - which is the currently used system in the majority of the laboratories - are questionable. It may be argued, however, that the use of orthotopically transplanted tumours is not feasible for a large-scale screening programme, being technically difficult and too expensive. In the case of ovarian carcinoma, the natural location of the tumour spread is the peritoneal cavity and it is therefore interesting to obtain tumour xenografts growing in the peritoneal cavity and forming ascites and metastatic deposits in the peritoneal organs [17,18]. Some of these tumours are currently used for testing drugs, after being validated with known drugs. For example, it has recently been seen that taxol is effective against human ovarian carcinoma growing in the peritoneal cavity of nude mice, even when derived from patients resistant to cisplatinum [19], a finding consistent with the clinical data on taxol activity in refractory ovarian cancer.

In some cases repeated human tumour biopsies from the same patient, taken at different times during the national history of the disease (e.g. at the first surgery before any chemotherapy, after relapse or progression following chemotherapy) can be successfully transplanted into nude mice [18]. These are unique and potentially useful models to investigate new drugs which may be effective in resistant tumours or are designed to circumvent drug resistance.

It is obvious that a very complete biological and pharmacological characterisation of xenografts appears necessary in order to select the optimal tumour xenograft to be used for a given compound, particularly when the mechanism of action and the pattern of cross-resistance have already been investigated in a simpler experimental model.

Other potentially interesting *in vivo* experimental models are transgenic and gene knock-out mice. These have certainly been extremely useful to elucidate the molecular mechanisms of carcinogenesis. To our knowledge no studies have been carried out so far on the use of these mice for the identification or evaluation of a *new* drug. For example transgenic mice with an activated *ras* gene [20] or altered expression of *erb-ß2* [21] have been described, but their employment for drug testing appears still to be at an early stage.

Other interesting *in vivo* models are those xenografts which derive from tumours with a specific genetic abnormality. Some human leukaemias and lymphomas are now well characterised from a molecular point of view [22]. Some translocations, such as the t(9,22) which gives rise to the fusion gene *bcr-abl* in CML and in some ALL; the translocation t(14,18) in B cell lymphoma where a *bcl-2*/immunoglobulin gene fusion is formed, or the t(15,17) in acute promyelocitic leukaemia (APL) where the genes for the retinoic acid receptor (RAR-α) and the

zinc finger protein PML become fused, are now established. It appears possible to obtain cell lines of these leukaemias [23], transplanted in SCID mice and maintaining the same rearrangements and translocations of the leukaemia or lymphoma they derive from [24]. These lines are obviously very useful to identify new drugs specifically active against these types of haematological malignancies. In addition, the fusion genes contain a chimeric DNA sequence uniquely present in these leukaemia cells, which represents an ideal target for antisense or antigene therapies as well as for DNA-sequence specific drugs [22, and see the first two chapters of the previous ESO Monograph *New Approaches in Cancer Pharmacology: Drug Design and Development*].

Conclusions

The selection of optimal experimental models for identifying and testing new anticancer agents is still an unsolved crucial issue. Our improved knowledge of tumour biology has increased the possibility of identifying cellular molecules which are, theoretically, suitable targets for novel drugs. Insufficient effort has so far been made to develop adequate *in vitro* and *in vivo* models to test drugs acting on specific targets. Here we have discussed the potential limitations of both the old and the new evaluation systems and indicated some possible ideas for future development.

Considering the high degree of heterogeneity of human tumours, it may be predicted that in order to be able to adequately represent the wide variety of human cancers, many different experimental models will be needed. Genetically manipulated and/or molecularly well characterised systems will certainly be useful to identify drugs selective for certain tumour types. It is envisaged that during the next years the exciting discoveries on the biology of human tumours will be accompanied by a parallel development of new experimental models to specifically test innovative therapeutic approaches.

DNA complexes of the two molecules, although there is as yet no direct evidence for this occurring. Molecular structural data on the enzyme is not yet available; it may well then be possible to rationally design more effective inhibitors of the enzyme-DNA complex than those currently available. However, there is little evidence of qualitative differences in primary sequence (and hence tertiary structure) in topoisomerase II between normal and tumour cells that could be exploited by rational drug design, apart from differences implicated in drug resistance mechanisms. It is thus unlikely that future X-ray crystallographic determination of the 3-dimensional structure of DNA topoisomerase II or its component sub-units, will lead to compounds specific to tumour cells, even though such data will certainly lead to a greater understanding of its role at the molecular level.

The large body of knowledge now available on oncogene sequences provides specific DNA targets that chemotherapy should in principle be able to exploit in order to down-regulate and suppress the expression of oncogenic proteins. This chapter examines the various approaches to the rational design of such highly specific agents, emphasising the role of molecular structural principles in the design process. It has to be borne in mind that single-oncogene targeting has not yet proved to be a viable approach to chemotherapy; the overwhelming majority of human cancers are multi-factorial in origin, with multiple oncogenic events contributing to tumour growth and metastasis. It is thus important that an oncogene-targeted approach to a particular human cancer take into account not only the roles played by the major oncogenes and their gene products, but their inter-relationships. Our increasing knowledge of signal transduction pathways is especially important in this regard; oncogenes, growth factors or kinases that control important cascades of events in the cell cycle are prime candidates for intervention.

Perhaps the most straightforward category where a single molecular lesion is the direct causative event of human disease, is the leukaemias where chromosomal breaks result in translocations of genes between chromosomes. The uncontrolled expression of gene products from these translocations can be directly correlated with disease. In chronic myelogenous leukaemia, the Philadelphia chromosome is generated by translocation of the *abl* gene on chromosome 9 to the *bcr* (breakpoint cluster region) gene on chromosome 22; the resulting *bcr-abl* hybrid gene product is identifiable as the overwhelming factor associated with blast-phase disease [5]. Its gene is therefore an excellent target for nucleic acid sequence-specific drugs that would inhibit its transcription/translation and expression of the *bcr-abl* protein [6]. The facile distribution of drugs in haematological cancers compared to solid tumours is a further reason for using the former as a test-bed for DNA-informational drugs since distribution problems would be minimised. Already, *ex-vivo* trials are planned in a number of centres on bone marrow from chronic myelogenous leukaemia patients, using anti-sense oligonucleotides to *bcr-abl* mRNA sequences.

Requirements for DNA Sequence Specificity

True specificity for a unique DNA site, in terms of the length of the human genome (about 3.5×10^9 base pairs), can only be achieved with a ligand that recognises at least 16-20 consecutive base pairs [7]. This range of lengths is calculated on the basis of a statistically random distribution of nucleotides in the genome (Table 1), with $(4^n)/2$ sites for an odd number n of base pairs, and $(4^n)/2 + (4^{n+2})/2$ for even n. This assumes an equal number of AT and GC

Table 1. The probability of finding a probe DNA sequence n base pairs long, expressed as the length of sequence in which n occurs uniquely

n	Length of unique sequence
2	10
3	32
4	136
5	512
6	2080
7	8192
8	32896
9	131072
10	524800
12	8390656
15	536870912
16	2147516416

base pairs, as well as randomness in their distribution. If the ratio AT:GC is not unity (which overall it is not in the human genome), then the minimum length required of the recognition oligonucleotide differs depending on whether it is purely AT or GC-containing. It is clearly advisable to verify the actual unique occurrence of a particular target sequence by systematic searching through a DNA databank, even though only a small fraction of the total genome is as yet sequenced. The under-representation of the dinucleotide sequence CpG is well documented, and can be straightforwardly taken into account in calculations such as those outlined above. This sequence has only about 20% of its random expected frequency in the overall genome, yet is over-represented in "CpG islands" in some housekeeping genes. It is not known if longer sequences have a non-random distribution in the genome - there may be biological and structural reasons for this being so. There have been recent findings that probes of 15 nucleotides in length are insufficient as human genome probes, and it has been suggested that lengths of 30-50 bases are required for true uniqueness [8].

Target oncogenic sequences can be one of a number of functional types. Some examples are given below that illustrate a diversity of potential therapeutic strategies and goals, ranging from the total shut-down of the expression of a particular gene, to diminution in over-expression, or the differentiation between a cellular gene required for normal cell growth, and its single point mutation [5]:

(i) a cellular proto-oncogene with point mutations that result in transforming properties, for example, the c-Ha-*ras* oncogene mutated at codons 12 or 61. Another important example is the p53 tumour suppressor gene, with transforming mutations at a large number of positions. In these circumstances, a high degree of discrimination at the DNA level would be required between the normal target sequence and where there is a single nucleotide change, of at least several orders of magnitude in binding affinities.

(ii) a cellular oncogene whose over-expression can lead to transforming properties. Examples are the nuclear oncogenes c- and N-*myc*, which occur in a wide variety of tumours and whose amplification can often be correlated with disease state, and the *erb*B genes coding

for transmembrane tyrosine kinases, which are frequently associated with breast carcinomas.

(iii) an oncogene produced by chromosomal translocation. Examples are the Philadelphia *bcr-abl* translocation in chronic myelogenous leukaemia, and the c-*myc* translocation to immunoglobin loci in Burkitt's lymphoma.

DNA-binding agents that are designed to be specific for sequences in the genes (exons or introns) of these targets, do require assays that reflect this functionality. Classic cytotoxicity testing, or even the more recent disease-oriented screens at the National Cancer Institute, USA, are much less relevant, at least in the first instance. However, since the majority of human tumours are multi-factorial in origin and involve the complex interplay of several oncogenic factors, disease-oriented screens will undoubtedly play a significant role in subsequent development of these new agents as drugs. Thus, one can envisage a succession of screens being required, to initially assay for activity against a singular molecular target *in vitro* and *in vivo*, then against cell and xenograft lines for which the target has established relevance, and finally against transplanted tumours, again for which there is functional evidence linking the target gene to tumour growth (see also chapter by D'Incalci).

In principle, sequence-specific drugs can be targeted to several distinct regions on a gene. The nature of the ultimate biological response produced by such a drug is in part dependent on this factor. The information encoded in a given intronic DNA sequence is read by a number of regulatory proteins and transcription factors in order for transcription to be regulated and initiated, when coding exons are then transcribed by RNA polymerase. Although it is attractive at first sight to target regulatory regions, this does require such competing drugs to bind to DNA with very high affinities, greater than 10^{12}. Blockage of the precessing of polymerase along a sequence is probably easier to achieve, as is evidenced by the ability of some intercalating agents (with affinities in the 10^6 range) to do so, at least *in vitro* and at relatively high concentrations. The problem of accessibility to eukaryotic DNA through the nucleoprotein complex is probably not a severe one, since it has to become at least partially locally dissociated for transcription to occur [9].

Molecular Structural Aspects of DNA Sequence Recognition

The DNA double helix broadly retains its classic Watson-Crick B form in eukaryotic cells, even in chromatin. The two anti-parallel phosphodiester strands produce two helical indentations in the helix surface. These are the major and minor grooves, which differ substantially in their widths (11.7Å vs. 5.7Å for canonical sequence-averaged B-DNA). Extensive crystallographic studies on oligonucleotide sequences have shown that DNA structure itself is sequence-dependent, with variability being found in such features as intra-strand phosphate-phosphate distances, intra-strand base-base orientation and groove widths [10]. As yet, it is not possible to define general rules governing the relationships between primary sequence and detailed micro-structure, although sufficient

data are now available on particular sequences involved in AT tracts [11-13], so that some general conclusions can be drawn about them. The sequence-dependence of DNA structure, flexibility and electronic properties are major factors in determining sites of protein and ligand binding. Molecules that interact with DNA other than purely at the phosphate groups, access the atoms and groups of the purine and pyrimidine bases via these grooves, and the size of their interacting groups relative to groove width is itself of importance in determining accessibility to bases involved in direct DNA recognition. Some years ago, prior to any molecular structural information on DNA-binding proteins, it was suggested [14] that sequence information is completely available as patterns of hydrogen bonding on the nucleotide bases, over and above Watson-Crick hydrogen-bonding (Fig. 1). Protein-DNA recognition would then involve direct readout of these differences in pattern on precessing along the helix or binding to a DNA sequence. Even at the single base-pair level, hydrogen bonding in the major groove can differentiate between AT and GC base pairs, with the former having an (acceptor,acceptor,donor) pattern and the latter being (acceptor, donor,acceptor). Discrimination between GC and CG is also possible on this basis. On the other hand, the minor groove is less rich in hydrogen-bonding potential, with an AT base pair being equivalent to a TA one since both have an (acceptor,acceptor) pattern. A GC base pair in the minor groove is distinguished from an AT one by the extra hydrogen donating potential of the exocyclic N2 amino group of guanine, although again the CG and GC base pairs have a symmetrical pattern of hydrogen-bonding potential, with (acceptor, donor,acceptor). The narrowness of the minor groove precludes all three of the GC hydrogen bonds being recognised, and in reality the width, especially in AT regions, only allows for one hydrogen bond per base. The geometric relationships between these donor and acceptor groups on successive bases in a sequence are invariant in an exactly repetitive double helix. However, sequence-dependent structural features in DNA structure will necessarily alter these relationships. For example, the distance between successive adenine N6 donor groups is 3.5Å in canonical DNA and 3.3Å for the first two adenines in the crystal structure of the sequence d(CGCGAATTC

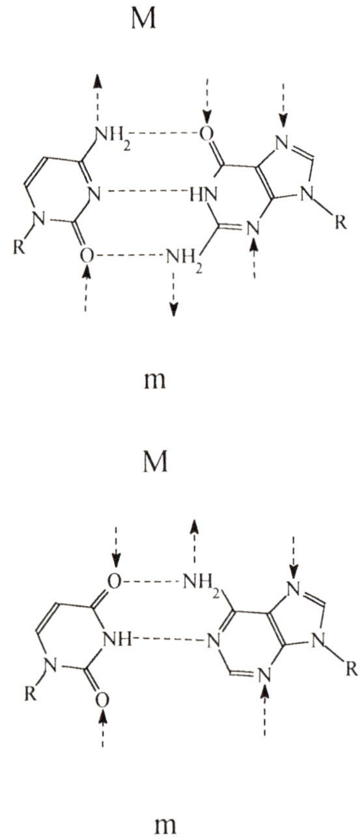

Fig. 1. Hydrogen bonding in a GC base pair (top) and an AT base pair (bottom). The major and minor groove sides are designated M and m, respectively. The direction of hydrogen-bond acceptance and donation to and from sites on the bases are shown by dotted arrows.

GCG)$_2$, which is the best-studied example of a sequence-dependent oligonucleotide structure [15]. Such differences have a major consequence for sequence-dependent protein recognition by amino-acid side-chains. The pattern of interactions seen in a particular protein-DNA complex is only applicable to the structural and dynamic properties of that DNA sequence. Others will require a quite distinct pattern of amino-acid side-chains. This need for precise geometric relationships between successive base pairs is seen in the features of arginine side-chains bridging, via hydrogen bonding, the N7 atoms of adjacent adenine bases in the crystal structure of the Eco RI-DNA endonuclease complex [16].

A number of distinct DNA-recognising structural motifs, such as helix-turn-helix [17], zinc finger [18], ß-sheet [19] or helix/ß barrel [20], have now been found by X-ray crystallographic analyses of DNA-binding proteins [21], often complexed with their oligonucleotide consensus sequences. Undoubtedly, more remain to be discovered. The helix-turn-helix pattern, which is found in a wide range of regulatory proteins from bacterial and mammalian sources, involves an α-helix interacting in a DNA major groove, and held in position by a second α-helix, with a tight ß-turn between them. The protein-DNA interactions found in the structures of the *cro* and 434 bacterial repressor complexes and the eukaryotic homeodomain repressor MATα2 show patterns of hydrogen-bonding involving such a recognition helix, although there is very limited consistency between the patterns [21,22]. The homeodomain structure actually has only three major-groove hydrogen bonds between protein and DNA, with a consensus binding site that is 9 base pairs long. Thus, direct DNA sequence readout by the protein via hydrogen bonding is only one contributor to total sequence-specific recognition. The other factor is presumed to be DNA structure itself, with its sequence-dependent structural and dynamic features being recognised as subtle differences in phosphodiester backbone conformation - this has been termed indirect DNA readout. Extensive interactions with backbone phosphate groups have been documented for the homeodomain-DNA complexes [17,23] and for the bacterial *trp* repressor [24]. There have been numerous attempts to define generalised amino acid-DNA recognition codes, largely based on principles of simple hydrogen-bonding direct readout; it is now clear that, at least for helix-turn-helix proteins, such a code cannot be straightforward and will remain elusive until considerably more is known about the way in which DNA structure controls indirect readout.

The DNA Minor Groove - a Target for Inhibitors of Transcription?

Until recently, the minor groove of DNA was considered to be unimportant for protein-DNA recognition, except possibly for non-specific interactions involving highly basic proteins such as the histones. This was attributed to the inherently decreased ability for minor groove direct sequence readout compared to the major groove. This picture has now changed. In the case of the homeodomains, their N-termini have been found in the crystal structures of their DNA complexes to be interacting in the minor groove of AT regions of the binding sequences [17,23], with arginine side-chains hydrogen-bonding to base atoms O2 of thymine and/or N3 of adenine. It has been suggested that the general motif SPKK (serine/threonine-proline-lysine/arginine-lysine/arginine), which is found as a repeating motif in histone H1 and in the HMG family of proteins [25], binds in the minor groove, presumably in a similar manner. The HMG box has been discovered in a number of transcription factors and sex-determining proteins [26] and appears to be an important DNA-regulatory structural type; as yet there is no detailed molecular structural information on it.

The key role played by minor groove recognition in gene regulation has recently been revealed by studies on the transcription factor TFIID. The conserved sequence TATA is the recognition point for the initiation of transcription by RNA polymerase in eukaryotic cells, and is ca. 30 base pairs upstream of the transcription start point. TFIID specifically binds to this sequence, as a key member of the group of general transcription factors [27] that assemble together around the TATA site and form a target site for upstream gene-specific promotors. TFIID has been shown by chemical protection studies [28,29] to bind at the TATA locus through the minor groove, possibly utilising a ß-sheet motif [30]. Even non-covalent binding drugs such as distamycin can effectively compete for this type of site, as least in the home-odomain regulatory proteins [31], so it is tempting to speculate that strong drug binding/bonding to the 4 base pairs of TATA and consequent inhibition of TFIID interaction, can be an effective means of transcription inhibition in those tumour cells that are actively proliferating. It is significant that the TFIID protein has recently been found to be over-expressed in human lung and breast carcinoma [32].

DNA Minor Groove Binders as Drugs

There are currently two principal approaches to the development of synthetic anti-gene agents. One uses defined-sequence oligonucleotides directed against either mRNA or against double-stranded DNA itself (the anti-sense and triplex anti-gene strategies). Their relative merits and de-merits have been described in detail elsewhere [49]. We focus instead on the alternative approach, which is concerned with the design and synthesis of semi and totally synthetic DNA-recognising (information-reading) molecules. The foregoing discussion has emphasised the roles played by regulatory proteins in gene transcription. By implication, inhibitory ligands need to effectively compete with them if they are to have a significant effect. This highlights a current major advantage of the non-oligonucleotide approach: both anti-sense and antigene oligonucleotides bind only relatively weakly to single and double-stranded nucleic acids, and hence are required in very considerable excess. The DNA-binding potency of synthetic DNA-reading molecules, by contrast, can be very high and moreover readily altered.

The starting points for these molecules have been on the one hand non-covalently binding anti-viral and cytotoxic agents such as the natural products netropsin and distamycin (which select AT sequences), and on the other the covalently-bonding anti-tumour agents anthramycin and CC1065 (which interact with N2 of guanine and N3 of adenine, respectively). Both classes of molecule bind in the minor groove of DNA and recognise up to 4-5 base pairs. To date, no analogous families of major-groove binding and reading molecules have been found or devised; the majority of alkylating agents such as the nitrogen mustards, methylating agents and cis-platinum all

interact with major-groove sites (typically the O6 or N7 base atoms), but do not actually read any sequence information. These agents would be expected to generally inhibit major-groove binding proteins such as the helix-turn-helix family. DNA repair mechanisms, which are induced by aberrations in DNA structure, will therefore be more important in the case of major-groove alkylation such as that of cis-platinum (which produces major distortions and bends DNA by 35-45° as a necessary consequence of intra-strand guanine cross-linking), than for minor-groove binding. The antibiotic CC1065 has high specificity to sequences such as 5'-AAAAA and induces bending of 17-22°, which is comparable to that found in natural AT tracts [33,34]. Thus, minor-groove binding drugs should have superior persistence on DNA in a biological sense as a result of their inherent shape complementarity to the minor groove and consequent minimal distortion of standard B-DNA.

Structural Aspects of Minor Groove Drug-DNA Complexes

Non-Covalent Complexes

Crystallographic studies have been reported on a number of minor-groove drug complexes with oligonucleotides [35], which provide detailed pictures of the recognition processes involved. All of these crystal structures (some 12 in all) involve non-covalent complexes with dodecanucleotide duplexes of the general type d(CGCPu(A/T)(A/T)(A/T)(A/T)PyGCG)$_2$.

The AT stretches have been 5'-AATT, 5'-AAATTT or 5'-ATATAT, thereby representing various types of AT tract. The drugs studied in these complexes have included distamycin, netropsin, pentamidine and berenil (Fig. 2), all of which have been shown by biophysical and footprinting analyses to bind to AT-rich sequences. As yet, no crystal structure of a covalent complex has been reported, although a number of nuclear magnetic resonance analyses have provided important structural information on them. In general, the crystal structures have all shown that the drugs bind in the AT-rich minor groove regions of the sequences,

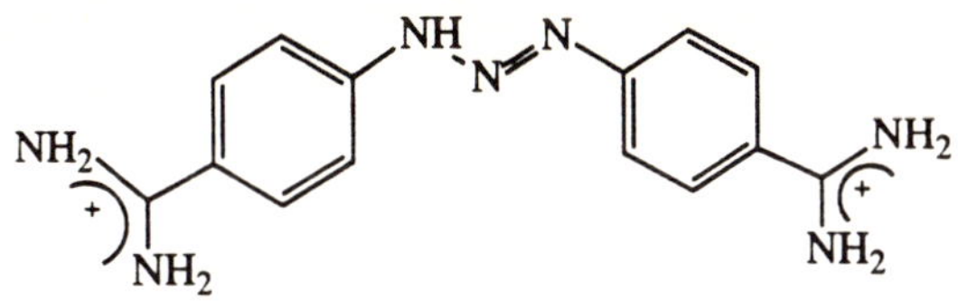

Berenil

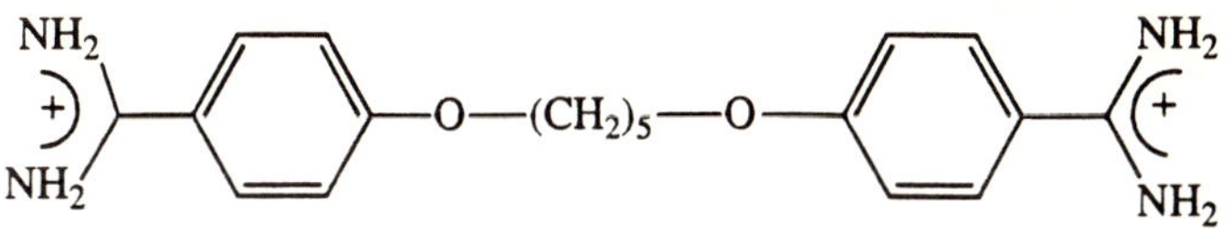

Pentamidine

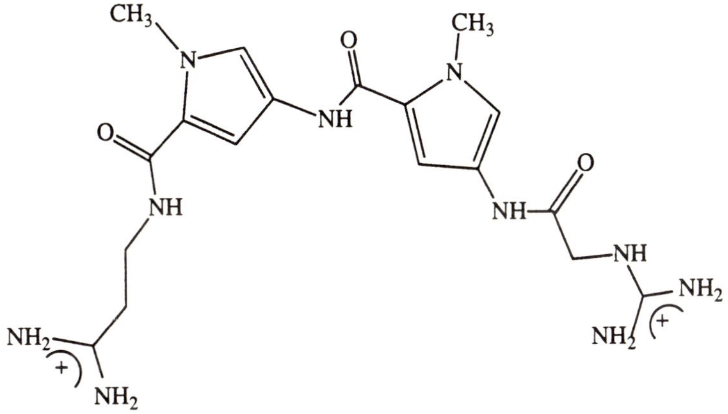

Netropsin

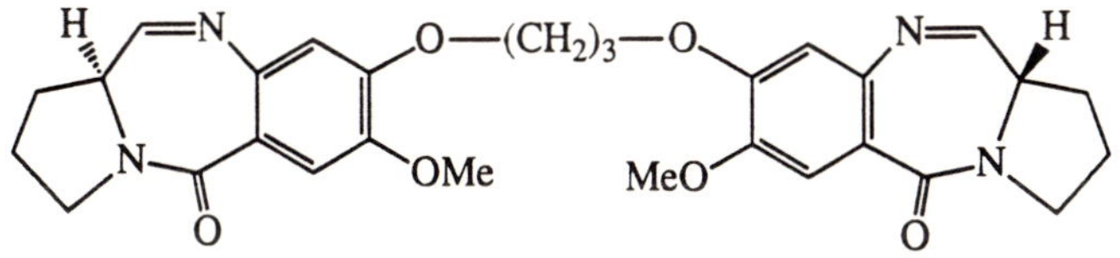

DSB-120

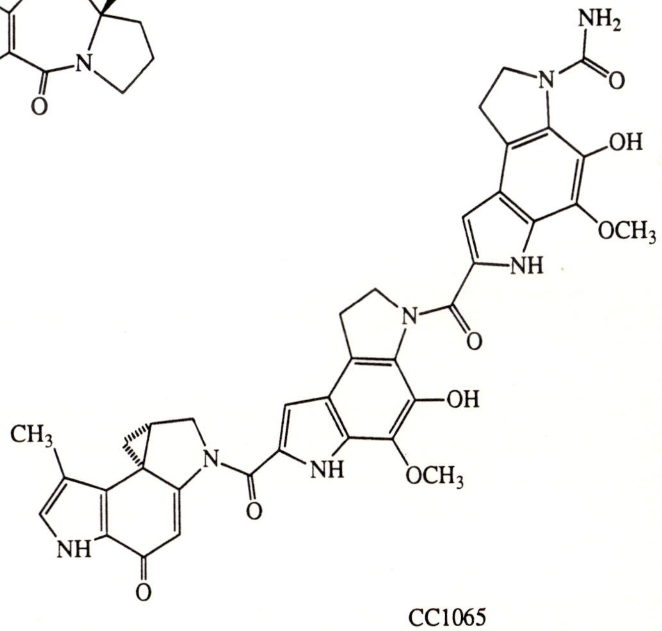

CC1065

Fig. 2. Structures of some minor groove-binding drugs

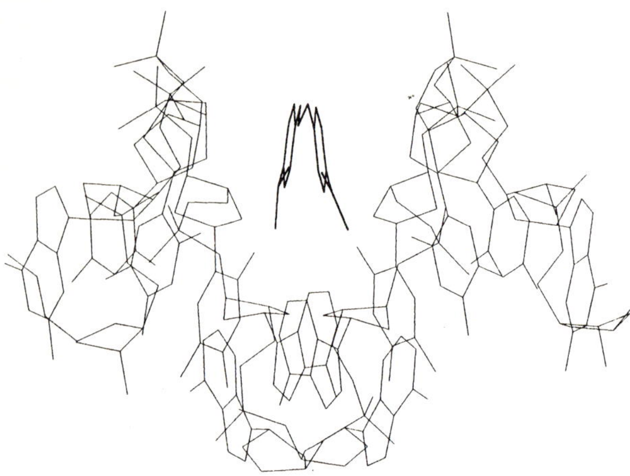

Fig. 3. A computer-drawn view of the structure of the berenil complex with the sequence d(CGCGAATTCG CG)₂, looking down the minor groove. The drug molecule is in bold outline.

with typically the minor groove itself being much narrower than in standard B-DNA. Hydrogen bonding has been observed in all of the complexes, between donor groups on the drug molecules and the minor-group acceptor atoms on adenine (N3) or thymine (O2) bases. The conformations of the oligonucleotides in these complexes barely change on drug binding, with, for example, the 5'-AAATTT sequence in its berenil complex [36] having the same pattern of base-pair sequence-dependent features as the drug-free sequence [11]. This has a number of features that resemble those of a long AT tract, especially those concerned with sequence-dependent base-pair geometry, such as propeller twist and roll. It is notable that the values of these parameters at several points along the 5'-AAATTT sequence differ from those in the corresponding berenil complex involving a 5'-AATT central sequence [37]. These differences have the effect of forcing a major change in the manner that berenil is bound to the AT region in one complex compared to another, and altogether demonstrate the inter-relationship between DNA sequence and structure. Thus, in the berenil complex involving the 5'-AAATTT sequence, there are hydrogen bonds between the terminal amidinium groups of the drug and thymine O2 atoms, from thymines 2 and 5, the drug thus occupying a 4 base pair site. In the 5'-AATT complex, hydrogen bonds are to N3 atoms of adenines 2 and 4, with the drug-base hydro-

gen bond being mediated through a water molecule; here the drug-binding site is 3 base pairs long. These analyses of berenil complexes indicate that this drug has a preference for 5'-pupuATTpy sequences, showing that flanking sequences play a role in determining the major binding site.

The structural studies outlined above have revealed that factors other than generalised electrostatic interactions and direct sequence readout by directional hydrogen-bonding are significant contributors to the recognition of AT sequences. In particular, the drugs have pronounced hydrophobic groupings (for example the phenyl rings in berenil and pentamidine), which are in close contact with the hydrogen atoms attached to the phosphodiester backbone that are concentrated at the opening of the minor groove (Fig. 3). These hydrophobic interactions serve to maintain the drug in an optimal position within the minor groove and can only occur when the groove is sufficiently narrow. They thus provide an effective mode of indirect sequence readout. AT-rich sequences such as 5'-AATT appear to have optimal width for these hydrophobic interactions, with very similar widths of the drugs and the minor groove. Other AT sequences have wider minor grooves and their flexibility is insufficient for narrowing and hence for effective binding to take place. Detailed mapping of drug-DNA nonbonded distances for both berenil and pentamidine [38,39] has shown that it is possible to ascribe distinct interaction functionality to different regions of the drug molecules (Fig. 4). This mapping can enable the design of analogues with altered binding properties to be performed in a rational manner [40].

Covalent Complexes

Heroic and extensive efforts have been made to switch the non-covalent recognition shown by the distamycins and netropsin from purely AT to more general mixed sequences involving GC base pairs. These have been based on the principle of replacing a hydrogen-bond donor group in these drugs by an acceptor, so as to interact with the N2 substituent atom of guanine [41]. However, it appears that this type of strong non-covalent binding in the minor groove is inextricably linked to AT sequences. A number of compounds in the lexitropsin series of ligands, which are based on netropsin, do show a degree of GC recognition, but overall strength of binding is invariably significantly less than that of the parent compound. A major factor in the reduction of binding affinity is undoubtedly the marked sequence dependence of minor-groove width. DNA regions with GC base pairs have wide minor grooves, with for example that in the sequence 5'-AGCT having a width of ~6.5Å compared to ~3.5Å for 5'-AATT [42]. Thus, effective hydrophobic interactions cannot occur and the diminished GC recognition is thus unsurprising. The recent finding [43] of specific binding to the sequence 5'-TGACT by the sterically wide dimer of the 1-methylimidazole-2-carboxamide derivative of netropsin, is a further demonstration of the importance of groove width in sequence recognition, and a possible pointer to a new type of minor-groove information readout.

Active GC recognition can be achieved very much more readily when drug binding involves covalent bonding to N2 of guanine, as occurs with the anthramycin family of compounds [1]. Anthramycin itself is only a modest DNA binder/bonder, and shows a preference for 5'-puGpu motifs. A C8-linked dimer of anthramycin, with a flexible -O-(CH$_2$)$_3$-O- linker, has recently been developed [44]. This compound (DSB120; Fig. 2) forms irreversible inter-strand cross-links, unlike anthramycin itself. Molecular modelling and nuclear magnetic resonance studies have shown that it binds to a 6 base-pair site of sequence 5'-puGATCpy. DSB120 is cytotoxic at the sub-nanomolar level to tumour cell lines *in vitro*. DNA-binding, cross-linking efficiency and cytotoxicity are correlated with linker chain length, with even numbers of methylene groups showing reduced effectiveness.

Several other minor-groove covalently-binding molecules are currently under active development as potential anticancer agents. All form covalent links with N3 of adenine, and do not appear to be extending sequence recognition beyond purely AT sequences. Carzelesin is a CC1065 analogue with the structural features that contribute to the "delayed death" properties of the parent compound having been designed out. It is cytotoxic at the nanomolar level and shows significant experimental antitumour activity [45]. It is in early clinical trial, as is the mustard derivative of distamycin (FCE24517)

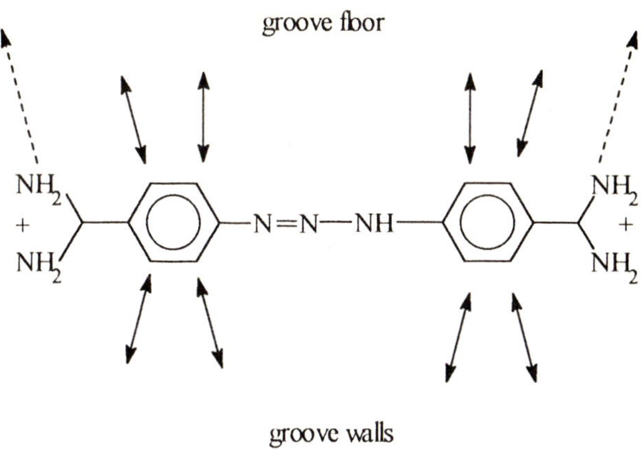

Fig. 4. Schematic of the various interactions between berenil and the minor groove. The dotted arrowed lines indicate hydrogen bonding to N3 of adenine or O2 of thymine. The solid arrows indicate that the inner edges of the phenyl rings in the drug molecule are in close van der Waals contact with the floor of the minor groove, comprising the hydrophobic edges of the bases. The outer edges of the phenyl rings have extensive hydrophobic close contacts with the hydrophobic outer edges of the minor groove.

[46]. Mustard groupings have also been employed in a series of 4-anilinoquinoline anilines that have *in vitro* and *in vivo* activity [47].

Sequence Specificity and Biological Function

As yet, there are remarkably few data on the question of the molecular locus of biological action of the minor-groove drugs, and how their sequence-specificity as found *in vitro* relates to this. Undoubtedly, encouraging clinical data will provide an impetus to such studies. We have suggested here that binding to critical sites such as the TATA signal sequence will inhibit transcription and thus may be an important aspect of the action of drugs such as CC1065, carzelesin and distamycin. Covalent groove-binding molecules will undoubtedly be the most efficient inhibitors in terms of competing with regulatory proteins such as TFIID.

The extensive structural and solution data on minor-groove binding agents does show that they can be highly specific to certain sequences, primarily (though not exclusively) AT ones. The major question facing the future development of new compounds is whether they can be designed around any desired sequence and thus can be used to target the oncogene and other sequences outlined above. A solution to this problem will undoubtedly arise from the further application of structural information in a systematic manner. This should enable, for example, discrimination between different AT and even GC sequences on the basis of differing groove widths and complementary features of hydrophobicity as well as directed hydrogen bonding. The ability to specifically recognise GC base pairs is best achieved by covalent binding, with for example the anthramycin moiety of DSB120 being such a recognition element. It is not difficult to envisage the assembly of these AT and GC-sensing elements together in order to read >12 base pairs by a combination of direct and indirect DNA readout.

Acknowledgements

I am grateful to the Cancer Research Campaign for their support of studies of drug-DNA recognition in my laboratory, and to many colleagues for discussion, especially David Thurston, Terry Jenkins and Charles Laughton.

REFERENCES

1   Hurley LH: DNA and associated targets for drug design. J Med Chem 1989 (32): 2027-2033
2   Lee HH, Palmer BD, Boyd M, Baguley C and Denny WA: Potential antitumour agents. 64. Synthesis and antitumour evaluation of dibenzo[1,4]dioxin-1-carboxamides: A new class of weakly binding DNA-intercalating agents. J Med Chem 1992 (35):258-266
3   Judson IR: Anthrapyrazoles: true successors to the anthracyclines? 1991 (2):223-231
4   Pommier Y, Capranico G, Orr A and Kohn WK: Distribution of topoisomerase II cleavage sites in simian virus 40 DNA and the effects of drugs. J Mol Biol 1991 (222):909-924
5   Vile RG (ed) Introduction to the Molecular Genetics of Cancer. John Wiley, Chichester 1992
6   Szcylik C, Skorski T, Nicholaides NC, Manzella L, Malaguarnera L, Venturelli D, Gewirtz AM and Calabretta B: Selective inhibition of leukemia cell proliferation by BCR-ABL antisense oligodeoxynucleotides. Science 1991 (253):562-565
7   Dervan PB: Design of sequence-specific DNA-binding molecules. Science 1986(232):464-471
8   Anderson C: NIH and DNA patent rejected; backers want to amend law. Nature 1992 (359):263
9   Felsenfeld G: Chromatin as an essential part of the transcriptinal mechanism. Nature 1992 (355):219-224
10 Dickerson RE: DNA structure from A to Z. Methods in Enzymology 1992 (211):67-111
11 Edwards KJ, Brown DG, Spink N, Skelly JV and Neidle S: Molecular structure of the B-DNA dodecamer d(CGCAAATTTGCG)$_2$. J Mol Biol 1992 (226):1161-1173
12 Yuan H, Quintana J and Dickerson RE: Alternative structures for alternating poly(dA-dT) tracts: The structure of the B-DNA decamer C-G-A-T-A-T-A-T-C-G. Biochemistry 1992 (31):8009-8021
13 Quintana JR, Grzeskowiak K, Yanagi K and Dickerson RE: Structure of a B-DNA decamer with a central T-A step: C-G-A-T-T-A-A-T-C-G. J Mol Biol 1992 (225):379-395
14 Seeman NC, Rosenberg JM and Rich A: Sequence-specific recognition of double helical nucleic acids by proteins. Proc Natl Acad Sci USA 1976 (73):804-808
15 Dickerson RE and Drew HR: Structure of a B-DNA dodecamer. II. Influence of base sequence on helix structure. J Mol Biol 1981 (149): 761-786
16 McClarin JA, Frederick CA, Wang B-C, Greene P, Boyer HW, Grable J and Rosenberg JM: Structure of the DNA-Eco RI endonuclease recognition complex at 3Å resolution. Science 1986 (234):1526-1541
17 Wolberger C, Vershon AK, Liu B, Johnson AD and Pabo CO: Crystal structure of a MATa2 homeodomain-operator complex suggests a general model for homeodomain-DNA interactions. Cell 1991 (67):517-528
18 Pavletich NP and Pabo CO: Zinc finger-DNA recognition: Crystal structure of a Zif268-DNA complex at 2.1Å. Science 1991 (252):809-817
19 Somers WS and Phillips SEV: Crystal structure of the *met* repressor-operator complex at 2.8Å resolution reveals DNA recognition by ß-strands. Nature 1992 (359): 387-393
20 Hegde RS, Grossman SR, Laimins LA and Sigler PB: Crystal structure at 1.7Å of the bovine papillomavirus-1 E2 DNA-binding domain bound to its DNA target. Nature 1992 (359):505-512
21 Freemont PA, Lane AN and Sanderson MR: Structural aspects of protein-DNA recognition. Biochem J 1991 (278):1-23
22 Pabo CO and Sauer RT: Transcription factors: Structural families and principles of DNA recognition. Annu Rev Biochem 1992 (61):1053-1095
23 Kissinger CR, Liu B, Martin-Blanco E, Kornberg TB and Pabo CO: Crystal structure of an engrailed homeodomain-DNA complex at 2.8Å resolution: A framework for understanding homeodomain-DNA interactions. Cell 1990 (63):579-590
24 Otwinowski Z, Schevitz RW, Zhang R-G, Lawson CL, Joachimiak A, Marmorstein RQ, Luisi BF and Sigler PB: Crystal structure of *trp* repressor/operator complex at atomic resolution. Nature 1988 (335):321-329
25 Churchill MEA and Travers AA: Protein motifs that recognize structural features of DNA. Trends in Biological Sciences 1991 (16):92-98
26 van de Wetering M and Clevers H: Sequence-specific interaction of the HMG box proteins TCF-1 and SRY occurs within the minor groove of a Watson-Crick double helix. The EMBO J 1992 (11):3039-3044
27 Pugh BF and Tjian R: Diverse transcriptional functions of the multisubunit eukaryotic TFIID complex. J Biological Chem 1992 (267):679-682
28 Lee DK, Horikoshi M and Roeder RG: Interaction of TFIID in the minor groove of the TATA element. Cell 1991 (67):1241-1250
29 Starr BD and Hawley DK: TFIID binds in the minor groove of the TATA box. Cell 1991 (67):1231-1240
30 Nash HA and Granston AE: Similarity between the DNA-binding domains of IHF protein and TFIID protein. Cell 1991 (67):1037-1038
31 Dorn A, Affolter M, Müller M, Gehring WJ and Leupin W: Distamycin-induced inhibition of homeodomain-DNA complexes. The EMBO J 1992 (11):279-286
32 Wada C, Kasai K, Kameya T and Ohtani H: A general transcription initiation factor, human transcription factor IID, overexpressed in human lung and breast carcinoma and rapidly induced with serum stimulation. Cancer Res 1992 (52):307-313
33 Lee C-H, Sun D, Kizu R and Hurley LH: Determination of the structural features of (+)-CC-1065 that are responsible for bending of DNA. Chem Res in Toxicology 1991 (4):203-213
34 Sun D and Hurley LH: Inhibition of T4 DNA ligase activity (+)-CC-1065: demonstration of the importance of the stiffening and winding effects of (+)-CC-1065 on DNA. Anti-Cancer Drug Design 1992 (7):15-36
35 Kopka ML and Larsen TA: Netropsin and the lexitropsins. The search for sequence-specific minor-groove-binding ligands. In: Propst CL and Perun TJ (eds) Nucleic Acid Targeted Drug Design. Marcel Dekker, Inc, New York 1992 pp 303-374

36   Brown DG, Sanderson MR, Garman E and Neidle S: Crystal structure of a berenil-d(CGCAAATTTGCG) complex. An example of drug-DNA recognition based on sequence-dependent structural features. J Mol Biol 1992 (226):481-490

37   Brown DG, Sanderson MR, Skelly JV, Jenkins TC, Brown T, Garman E, Stuart DI and Neidle S: Crystal structure of a berenil-dodecanucleotide complex: The role of water in sequence-specific ligand binding. EMBO J 1990 (9): 1329-1334

38   Neidle S: Minor-groove width and accessibility of B-DNA drug and protein complexes. FEBS 1992 (298):97-99

39   Edwards KJ, Jenkins TC and Neidle S: Crystal structure of a pentamidine-oligonucleotide complex: Implications for DNA-binding properties. Biochemistry 1992 (31):7104-7109

40   Bruice TC, Mei H-Y, He G-X and Lopez V: Rational design of substituted tripyrrole peptides that complex with DNA by both selective minor-groove binding and electrostatic interaction with the phosphate backbone. Proc Natl Acad Sci USA 1992 (89):1700-1704

41   Dwyer TJ, Geierstanger BH, Bathini Y, Lown JW and Wemmer DE: Design and binding of a distamycin A analog to d(CGCAAGTTGGC)·d(GCCAACTTGCG): Synthesis, NMR studies, and implications for the design of sequence-specific minor groove binding oligopeptides. JACS 1992 (114):5911-5919

42   Webster GD, Sanderson MR, Skelly JV, Neidle S, Swann PF, Li BF and Tickle IJ: Crystal structure and sequence dependent conformation of the A·G mis-paired oliognucleotide d(CGCAAGCTGGCG). Proc Natl Acad Sci USA 1990 (87):6693-6697

43   Mrksich M, Wade S, Dwyer TJ, Geierstanger BH, Wemmer DE and Dervan PB: Antiparallel side-by-side dimeric motif for sequence-specific recognition in the minor groove of DNA by the design peptide 1-methylimidazole-2-carboxamide netropson. Proc Natl Acad Sci USA 1992 (89):7586-7590

44   Subhas Bose D, Thompson AS, Ching J, Hartley JA, Berardini MD, Jenkins TC, Neidle S, Hurley LH and Thurston DE: Rational design of a highly efficient non-reversible DNA interstrand cross-linking agent based on the pyrrolobenzodiazepine ring system. J Amer Chem Soc 1992 (114):4939-4941

45   Li LH, DeKoning TF, Kelly RC, Krueger WC, McGovren JP, Padbury GE, Petzold GL, Wallace TL, Ouding RJ, Prairie MD and Gebhard I: Cytotoxicity and antitumour activity of carzelesin, a prodrug cyclopropylpyrroloindole analogue. Cancer Res 1992 (52): 4904-4913

47   Fontana M, Lestingi M, Mondello C, Braghetti A, Montecucco A and Ciarrocchi G: DNA binding properties of FCE 24517, an electrophilic distamycin analogue. Anti-Cancer Drug Design 1992 (7):131-141

48   Gravatt, GL, Baguley BC, Wilson WR and Denny WA: DNA-directed alkylating agents. 4. 4-anilinoquinoline-based minor groove directed aniline mustards. J Med Chem 1991 (34):1552-1560

49   C. Hélène: Antisense and Antigene Oligonu-cleotides Targeted to Oncogenes. In: P. Workman (ed) New Approaches in Cancer Pharmacology: Drug Design and Development. European School of Oncology Monograph Series. Springer Verlag, Heidelberg 1992

Discovery of Improved Platinum Analogues

Kenneth R. Harrap

The Institute of Cancer Research: Royal Cancer Hospital, Drug Development Section, 15 Cotswold Road, Belmont, Sutton, Surrey SM2 5NG, United Kingdom

Background: Antitumour and Toxic Properties of Cisplatin

Although dichlorodiammine platinum II (Fig. 1) was first synthesised by Peyrone in 1845, the powerful antitumour properties (confined to the *cis*-isomer) remained unknown until the work of Barnett Rosenberg, some 125 years later. Rosenberg attributed the toxic effects of an alternating electric field applied to a suspension of *E. coli* to the generation of *cis*-dichlorodiammine platinum II (cisplatin). Subsequently, cisplatin was shown to possess potent activity, both alone and in combination, against a wide spectrum of transplantable rodent tumours [see 1-3 for reviews]. Preclinical toxicology was assessed in mice, rats, guinea pigs, dogs and monkeys and the results predicted well for those toxicities subsequently found in man [4]. Nephrotoxicity was the major dose-limiting side effect in all species, accompanied by gastrointestinal, haematological and ototoxicities, together with severe emesis in dogs and monkeys [5-11].
Cisplatin was shown to be very active in the treatment of testicular tumours, both alone and in combination with vinblastine and bleomycin [12-21]. It was also effective in ovarian cancer [22-25] and in bladder [26-29] and head and neck cancers [30, 31]. The toxicities predicted from the preclinical studies were encountered in man: nephrotoxicity remains the major dose-limiting side effect, though this can be ameliorated by intravenous hydration and diuresis [32-39]. Although this procedure facilitates the administration of higher doses of cisplatin, the incidence of other toxicities, notably deafness and peripheral neuropathy, is markedly in-creased [40]. Moderate to severe nausea and vomiting, which can be prolonged, is encountered frequently, together with tinnitus, hearing loss, peripheral neuropathy and myelosuppression [33-34, 41].
It is evident from this background that cisplatin is an exceptionally valuable, if exceptionally toxic, anticancer drug. Accordingly, much effort has been devoted to the discovery both of less toxic alternatives to cisplatin and of new platinum-based drugs which might possess activity in cisplatin-refractory and relapsed cancers.

Structural Requirements for Antitumour Activity

The reader is referred to [2] for a fuller elaboration of this topic. Space constraints permit only broad conclusions to be mentioned here. The greater majority of studies have concentrated on direct cisplatin analogues, that is, complexes of general type $[PtX_2A_2]$ where $X_2 =$

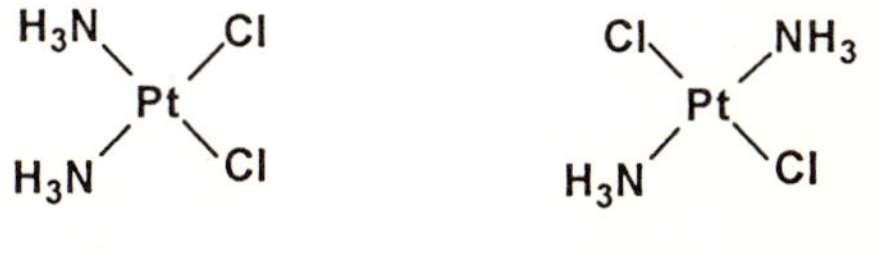

Fig. 1. Structures of cisplatin (*cis*-dichlorodiammine-platinum II) and transplatin (*trans*-dichloro *trans*-diammino platinum II)

two monodentate or one bidentate anionic ligand(s) and A_2 = two monodentate or one bidentate amine ligand(s). It is important to observe that much of the work on this topic has been dominated by *in vivo* antitumour evaluations in transplantable murine tumour models, such as those until only recently in use at NCI [3]. There is little opinion consensus that these models, which relied heavily on a mouse leukaemia prescreen, are representative either of human malignant diseases in man or of their response to chemotherapy. Indeed, NCI has now adopted a human disease-oriented screening strategy which is expected to be more predictive. This model consists of panels of well-characterised and calibrated (against drugs of established activity in man) human tumour cell lines in several disease categories [42]. As yet there is no information available from this model to confirm (or refute) the structure-activity indications which have been derived from studies with transplantable mouse tumours.

With this caveat in mind it is apparent that a primary requirement for antitumour activity is that the platinum coordination complex be uncharged, since polar molecules penetrate cell membranes with low efficiency. Both Pt(II) (square planar) and Pt(IV) (octahedral) complexes can possess antitumour properties, though the latter require reduction to the Pt(II) state in order to elicit biological activity. For both Pt(II) and Pt(IV) molecules, only those carrying *cis*-oriented ammine (A) and leaving group (X) ligands are endowed with antitumour (and toxic) properties: the corresponding *trans* isomers appear to be devoid of useful antitumour activities, though they can still initiate host toxicities. Molecules containing highly reactive leaving (X) groups, such as NO_3^- and H_2O are predominantly toxic, while those containing strongly bound ligands, such as SCN^- and NO_2^-, are biologically inert. Useful biological properties appear to be confined to molecules of intermediate stability containing Cl^- or Br^- ligands, Finally, it is apparent that unsubstituted *bis*-diammine ligands are not obligatory for activity. Both *bis*-diamines, non-symmetrically substituted diamines, or ammine/amines (so called "mixed amines") can possess antitumour properties. Frequently the latter are associated with increased selectivity, attributable largely to reduced host toxicities.

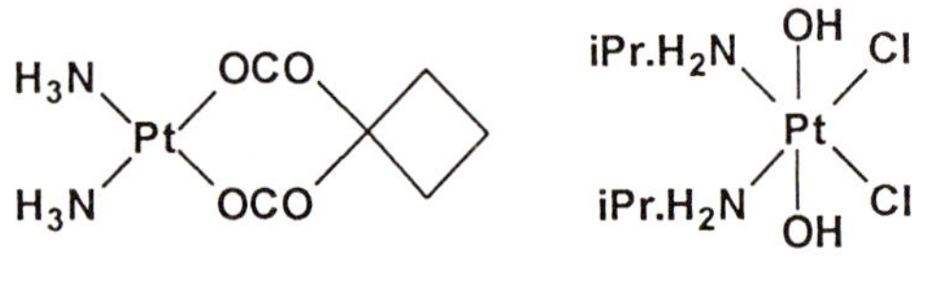

Major Preclinical "Leads"

Probably the greatest volume of synthetic effort occurred during the 1970s and transplantable murine tumour models were exploited to establish the structure-activity principles outlined above. By 1980 some 1055 platinum complexes had been screened at NCI, from which it was concluded that 3 compounds, JM74 (1,2-diaminocyclohexane (malonato) platinum (II), JM82(1,2-diaminocyclohexane (4-carboxyphthalato) platinum (II) and JM8 [diammine (1,1-cyclobutyldicarboxylato) platinum (II), carboplatin] could be considered as prime "leads" for early clinical evaluation [43]. It is interesting that the prioritising by NCI of a less toxic (more selective) cisplatin analogue (carboplatin) and of complexes which circumvented acquired resistance in murine models (JM74, JM82) encapsulated the two major themes of new platinum drug discovery and also confirmed the observations of other laboratories.

The Institute of Cancer Research in Sutton, in collaboration with the Johnson Matthey Technology Centre, had elaborated a substantial portfolio of platinum complexes, many with good activity in preclinical rodent tumour models. As already indicated above, it became apparent that potent antitumour complexes were generally chemically reactive and toxic compounds. Thus, anti-tumour selectivity could be divorced from potency and a structure-(nephro)toxicity study suggested that JM8 (carboplatin) and JM9 [*cis*-dichloro-*trans*-dihydroxybis(isopropylamine) platinum (IV)] were viable candidates for clinical evaluation (Fig. 2).

CARBOPLATIN (PARAPLATIN, JM8)   IPROPLATIN (JM9)

Fig. 2. Structures of carboplatin [diammine(1,1-cyclobutanedicarboxylato) platinum II] and iproplatin [*cis*-dichloro-*trans*-dihydroxybis(isopropylamine) platinum IV]: less toxic clinically active analogues of cisplatin

Fig. 3. Structures of JM74 [1,2-diaminocyclohexane (malonato) platinumII] and JM82 [1-2-diaminocyclohexane (4-carboxyphthalato) platinum II]. These compounds were selected for clinical study because they retained activity in acquired cisplatin-resistant mouse leukaemias.

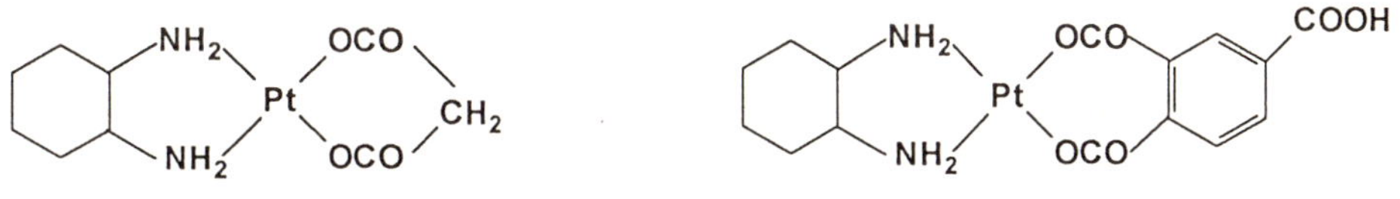

JM8 was preferred over JM9 because of superior biochemical and human tumour xenograft selectivity [5].

With separate objectives, Burchenal and colleagues were studying the structural requirements for circumvention of acquired cisplatin resistance in mouse leukaemia cell lines, both *in vitro* and *in vivo*. Whilst compounds effective in this model might be expected to possess activity in cisplatin-relapsed human disease (assuming that cisplatin (acquired) resistant leukaemias are predictive for relapsed disease in man), they could only be expected to be active in *ab initio* refractory human tumours if the mechanisms underlying both intrinsic and acquired resistance were identical. There is at present no evidence to suggest that this is the case. Nonetheless, Burchenal's work has provided an important stimulus to platinum drug discovery in the context of animal tumour models and their relevance to human disease. In essence, Burchenal and his group demonstrated that platinum complexes carrying either a 1,2-diaminocyclohexane or 1,2-diaminocycloheptane carrier ligand, regardless of the leaving groups, on a Pt(II) complex, failed to display cross-resistance with cisplatin in cisplatin-acquired resistant P388 and L1210 mouse leukaemias, both *in vitro* and *in vivo* [44-46]. In separate studies Schwartz et al. synthesised JM82 [1,2-diaminocyclohexane (4-carboxyphalato) platinum(II)] in an attempt to overcome the inherent aqueous insolubility of complexes carrying the 1,2-diaminocyclohexane ligand [47] such as JM74 [1,2-diaminocyclohexane (malonato)platinum II] (Fig. 3). This compound posessed broad spectrum activity in preclinical antitumour screens and received subsequent phase I/II clinical evaluation (see below).

These studies of 1,2-diaminocyclohexane complexes had been carried out mostly with racemates and Kidani et al. pointed to the existence of 3 isomeric forms incorporating *cis*, *trans-d* and *trans-l* isomers, corresponding to 1S, 2R; 1S, 2S and 1R, 2R configurations, respectively [48], each of which conferred quantitatively separate antitumour properties. Kidani was also responsible for the synthesis of oxaliplatin (*trans-l*) oxalato-1,2-diaminocyclohexane platinum(II) (see Fig. 4). This compound showed good activity in preclinical screening models and evidence of lack of cross-resistance with cisplatin in some acquired resistant cell lines [49-51]. The latest member of the group of platinum antitumour complexes carrying the 1,2-diaminocyclohexane ligand to undergo clinical study is tetraplatin, [(*trans-d,*) 1,2-diaminocyclohexanetetrachloro platinum (IV)] (see Fig. 4). It exhibits broad spectrum activity in preclinical antitumour screens, notably being non-cross-resistant with cisplatin in acquired resistant P388 and L1210 murine leukaemias [52]. The proximally active species *in vivo*, following reduction, is probably the corresponding Pt(II) complex [53,54]. Another Pt(II) complex containing the cyclohexane moiety [1,1-diaminomethylcyclohexane (sulphato) platinum(II), TNO6] was also found to be non-cross-resistant with cisplatin in the acquired resistant L1210 leukaemia [55]. The sulphate ligand is a reactive group which predisposes to nephrotoxicity (as was confirmed in a phase I study - see below).

Oxaliplatin (l-OHP)

Tetraplatin (Ormaplatin)

TN06

Predictive Utility of Screening Models

The advisability of relying heavily on mouse leukaemia screening models in platinum analogue development has been questioned by Goddard et al. [56]. These workers studied 2 tumour models, the L1210 and the ADJ/PC6 plasmacytoma, together with their cisplatin (acquired) resistant counterparts. It should be noted that the ADJ/PC6 plasmacytoma predicted well for the known clinical activity of cisplatin, carboplatin and iproplatin. When these 3 drugs, together with tetraplatin, were investigated it was found that the L1210/cisplatin-resistant tumour was cross-resistant also to carboplatin and iproplatin. However, tetraplatin proved to be even more active against the resistant L1210 than against the original "wild-type" tumour. On the other hand, the cisplatin-resistant ADJ/PC6 tumour was completely cross-resistant, not only to carboplatin and iproplatin, but also to tetraplatin. It is important that such predictive disparities in screening data be resolved by recourse to wider evaluation before a compound may be regarded with any confidence as a clinical development candidate. Accordingly, the group at the Institute of Cancer Research has concentrated on establishing in vitro and in vivo laboratory models of human ovarian cancer to further its new platinum drug discovery objectives. Ovarian cancer was targeted since this disease is sensitive to the 2 available registered platinum drugs (cisplatin and carboplatin). Response rates to either drug are approximately 50% and long-

term remissions can be achieved. However, the majority of responding patients eventually relapse, so the cure rate in this disease from platinum-based chemotherapy is exceptionally low. It is important therefore to have available models which are representative of both ab initio refractory disease (intrinsic resistance) and relapsed disease (acquired resistance). Human ovarian carcinoma cell lines have been established, characterised and calibrated against several platinum drugs. Acquired (cisplatin) resistant variants have also been developed, as have xenograft (nude mouse) counterparts of the in vitro lines. Thus realistic models are now available which permit structure-activity and mechanistic studies in tumour cell lines in vitro, together with related pharmacologic and toxicologic evaluations employing xenograft counterparts of the same cell lines in vivo [57-59]. When tetraplatin was studied in a panel of human ovarian carcinoma xenografts, activity was seen in only 2 of 16 tumours, neither of which was resistant to cisplatin. However, 7 xenografts were sensitive to both cisplatin and carboplatin [58].

Current Drug Development Initiatives

Ammine/Amine Complexes: Oral Drug Delivery

The benefits offered by this class of compounds in conferring enhanced tumour selectivity have already been mentioned. More recently the structure-activity relationships of such compounds have been investigated further in a panel of human ovarian carcinoma cell lines [60]. A particular advantage is conferred by the cyclohexylamine ligand in both platinum(II) and platinum(IV) complexes which are more potent than the corresponding unsubstituted parent *bis*-diamines. These findings have been exploited in the development of a new platinum drug designed for oral administration. Quality of life is an exceedingly important consideration in cancer chemotherapy. The availability of an oral platinum-based drug would be of considerable advantage in this context in the out-patient setting, simplifying dose administration and enabling schedule optimisation, whilst conferring associated benefits of cost-effectiveness.

A major initial problem proved to be the generally poor absorption of the majority of mixed amines evaluated. However, this difficulty was circumvented by the design and synthesis of a novel class of platinum(IV) ammine/amine dicarboxylate complexes of general formula $[c,t,c-\{PtCl_2(OCOR_1)_2NH_3(RNH_2)\}]$ [61]. These compounds are generally well absorbed from the gastrointestinal tract and possess *in vivo* oral activity in a wide range of murine and human tumour models [62,63]. The "lead" compound (JM216, $R_1=CH_3, R=cC_6H_{11}$) (Fig. 5) possesses oral activity comparable to systemically administered cisplatin and carboplatin in several murine tumours and human ovarian carcinoma xenografts. Toxicology studies in rodents show an absence of nephrotoxicity, with leucopenia being dose limiting [64]. JM216 is currently in phase I study in the Royal Marsden Hospital, Sutton and London.

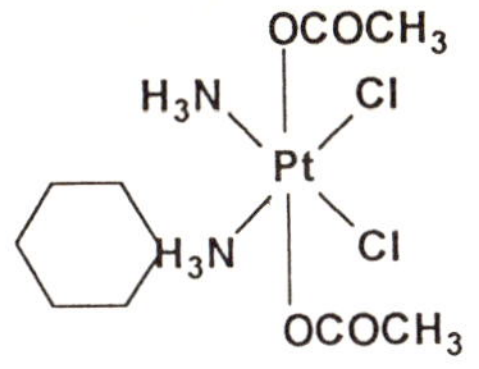

Improving Platinum Complex Uptake in Cisplatin-Resistant Cells

Acquired resistance to cisplatin has been attributed, classically, to several mechanisms, including impaired intracellular accumulation, enhanced intracellular detoxication (via elevated glutathione and/or metallothioneins) and enhanced repair, or tolerance, of DNA-platinum lesions [reviewed in 65-67]. Some of the mixed ammine/amines referred to above, where the axial dicarboxylate functions have been extended to contain 3 or more carbon atoms, are in excess of 100-fold more cytotoxic than cis-

OCOCH$_3$

H$_3$N   Cl

Pt

H$_3$N   Cl

OCOCH$_3$

JM216

Fig. 5. Structure of JM216 [*cis*-dichloro-*trans*-bis-acetato-*cis*-cyclohexylamine ammine platinum IV], a novel platinum IV coordination complex designed for oral administration

platin. Moreover, they retain cytotoxicity in cells which exhibit either acquired or intrinsic resistance to cisplatin primarily through impaired uptake of the drug [68,69]. Such compounds provide useful leads with which to elucidate the pharmacological requirements of platinum co-ordination complexes which circumvent transport-determined cisplatin resistance *in vitro*.

Altered Platinum-DNA Binding

Cisplatin and carboplatin produce similar spectra of DNA adducts, which presumably are removed and repaired by the same mechanisms [70]. In an attempt to design drugs which will bind to different loci on DNA, Farrell and co-workers have synthesised bis-platinum complexes in which 2 transplatin molecules are linked by an alkyl chain [71,72] (Fig. 6). The same group has also synthesised complexes containing bulky planar ligands such as pyridine or thiazole [73,74]. In a panel of human ovarian carcinoma cell lines the *trans*-$[PtCl_2(pyridine)_2]$ complex was comparably cytotoxic to cisplatin and retained activity in some cisplatin (acquired) resistant variants. Regrettably this promise has not been fulfilled *in vivo*, suggesting pharmacokinetic limitations in these structures [74].

Clinical Findings

Two broad structural themes have emerged from the preclinical development of cisplatin analogues. These relate to the separate objec-

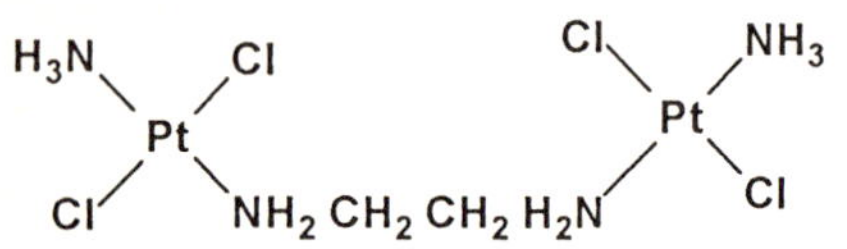

Fig. 6. Structures of bis-transplatin and *trans*-pyridine platinum II complexes which bind to different DNA loci from cisplatin

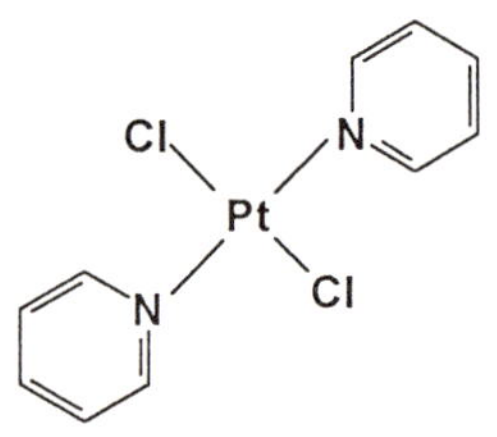

tives of (i) discovering compounds which circumvent cisplatin resistance, exploiting, predominantly, murine leukaemia screening models possessing acquired resistance to cisplatin, and (ii) discovering compounds which retain the useful antitumour properties of cisplatin, but which are better tolerated. The common structural feature of group (i) compounds is the presence of the 1,2-diaminocyclohexane ligand. Group (ii) compounds contain one or two carboxylate leaving groups, the majority being typified by the presence of the 1,1-cyclobutyldicarboxylate ligand. Such compounds are chemically more stable than cisplatin and are thus expected to be less toxic.

It is not intended, nor would it be appropriate, to provide a comprehensive review of all the platinum complexes which have been studied in the clinic to date. Rather it is the purpose to discuss those which confirm or refute preclinical drug design strategies and to comment briefly on some of the agents which are presently in the clinic.

Platinum Complexes Containing the 1,2-Diaminocyclohexane Ligand

1,2-diaminocyclohexane (malonato) platinum(II) (JM74)

This was the first of such complexes to be investigated [75-77]. Nausea and vomiting, se-

vere diarrhoea, leucopenia and thrombocytopenia were prominent side effects, though there was no evidence of nephrotoxicity. Some responses were seen, notably in AML. However, the limited solubility of this compound necessitated the infusion of prohibitively large volumes of fluid, such that dose-limiting toxicity was not achieved. There was no unambiguous indication of activity in cisplatin-refractory disease.

1,2-diaminocyclohexane (4-carboxyphthalato) platinum(II)

Phase I and II studies with this compound have been reported [78,79]. Dose-limiting toxicity was thrombocytopenia, though there was also evidence of nephrotoxicity. Nausea and vomiting occurred at all doses. There was also some concern at the incidence of peripheral neuropathy. Phase II studies included diseases normally sensitive to cisplatin and all patients had been previously treated with the drug. Of 8 patients with testicular cancer, no responses were seen, while one PR was observed in 8 patients with ovarian cancer. It must be concluded that this compound did not display the activity predicted for it in the preclinical studies.

Tetraplatin (ormaplatin)

Phase I studies are currently in progress on various schedules (q28d; d1 and d8q28d; dx5q28d) and only abstract reports are available [80-84]. Of most concern is the incidence of peripheral neuropathy which has been encountered in all studies, which may limit the further development of this compound. Emesis and myelosuppression have also been observed in all studies.

Oxaliplatin

Two conventional phase I studies have been reported, in both of which neurological toxicities (acute paraesthesia of the extremities, peripheral neuropathy) appeared to be dose limiting [85, 86]. Other toxicities were emesis, diarrhoea and myelosuppression. As yet there is no evidence for the activity of this drug against cisplatin-refractory disease in the phase II setting.

1,1-Diaminomethylcyclohexane(sulphato)platinum (II) (TNO6)

A single phase I study of this compound has been reported [87]. Of the 53 patients studied, most had received extensive prior treatment, including cisplatin. Dose-limiting toxicity was myelosuppression and renal failure. Proteinuria was observed when the drug was given by rapid infusion, though this could be restricted by extending the infusion time. Dose-related nausea and vomiting were observed in most patients, which in some could be controlled with conventional antiemetics. One complete response was seen in the lung metastases of a patient with breast cancer and a partial response in a patient with adenocarcinoma of the lung. All patients in the study were shown to be refractory to cisplatin, except for the patient with breast cancer. As with other drugs developed on the basis of activity against cisplatin-refractory mouse leukaemias, TNO6 fails to realise in the clinic the promise of the animal model predictions.

Platinum Complexes Containing Carboxylate Leaving Groups

Carboplatin (cis-diammine 1,1-cyclobutane dicarboxylato platinumII)

This drug has been registered world-wide and is clearly devoid of the major toxic limitations of cisplatin. Extensive discussion of its clinical development is inappropriate here and the reader is referred to recent review articles [88,89]. Randomised studies of carboplatin and cisplatin in ovarian cancer indicate comparable response and relapse rates [90,91]. Further, each drug appears to be active in the same patient population, and similar resistance mechanisms are presumably common to each drug [92,93]. In a randomised comparison of carboplatin and iproplatin [cis-dichloro-trans-di-hydroxy-bis(isopropylamine) platinum (IV)] in ovarian cancer, carboplatin appeared to possess better antitumour properties and less toxicity (in particular gastrointestinal and haematological) than iproplatin [94]. Thus it may be concluded that carboplatin is unquestionably a better tolerated drug than cisplatin but it has made no impact on the common problem of clinical resistance to the parent drug.

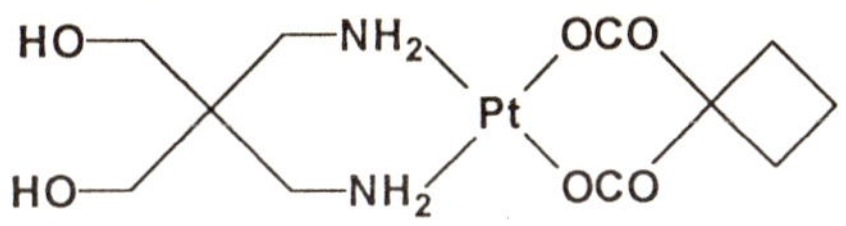

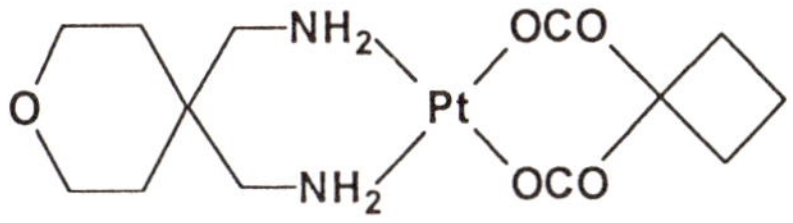

Fig. 7. Structures of zeniplatin and enloplatin

Zeniplatin and enloplatin

Zeniplatin and enloplatin (Fig. 7) are platinum(II) 1,1-cyclobutane dicarboxylates and as such are direct analogues of carboplatin. Both compounds were developed on the basis of activity in preclinical murine tumour screening models. In particular enloplatin [1,1-cyclobutanedicarboxylato(2-)-O,O'] (tetrahydro-4H-pyran-4,4-dimethanamine N,N') platinum(II)] possessed better activity than zeniplatin [2,2-bis(aminomethyl)-1,3-propanediol-N,N'] [1,1-cyclobutanedicarboxylato(2-)O,O']platinum(II) against the cisplatin acquired resistant L1210 leukaemia [95]. However, in two cisplatin-resistant human tumour cell lines zeniplatin was completely cross-resistant and enloplatin partially so [96]. Neither compound was nephrotoxic in the rat [95].

A phase I clinical study of zeniplatin has been reported [97]. The drug was given by 60- or 90-minute intravenous infusion every 21 days and doses escalated to a maximum tolerated dose of 145 mg/m^2. Dose-limiting toxicities were leucopenia and neutropenia. Emesis occurred at all doses above 50 mg/m^2, being severe in 50% of patients and non-responsive to low-dose oral metaclopramide. Notably a substantial fall in creatinine clearance (40%) was observed at the maximum tolerated dose. Three responses were observed.

A phase II study (bolus q21d) of zeniplatin in non-small cell lung cancer has been reported [98], while preliminary results have appeared of studies on the same schedule in melanoma [99,100], breast [101] and ovarian [102] cancers. A partial response rate of 22% was obtained in non-small cell lung cancer, comparable to that seen following cisplatin or carboplatin treatment. In the 2 ongoing melanoma studies a combined partial response rate of 19% has been obtained. Partial responses have also been observed in the ongoing breast and ovary trials. Major toxicities have been neutropenia and emesis, the latter being moderate or severe in at least 50% of patients despite prophylactic antiemetic therapy. An additional worrying feature has been the appearance of nephrotoxicity in all patients treated at 145 mg/m^2, despite intravenous hydration.

In a preliminary report of a phase I study of enloplatin (bolus q21d), neutropenia and leucopenia were observed at 1023 mg/m^2 and nephrotoxicity at 1227mg/m^2. The dose recommended for phase II study is 1023 mg/m^2 [103].

NK121(CI973) (cis-1,1-cyclobutanedicarboxylato(2R)-2-methyl-1,4-butanediamine-platinum(II))

This agent is one of two direct carboplatin analogues (the other is DWA2114R) in clinical development in Japan. It showed moderate activity in transplantable mouse tumour models and, unlike DWA2114R, is active in the L1210 cisplatin-resistant (acquired) leukaemia model [104]. Neutropenia was the dose-limiting toxicity at a (maximum tolerated) dose of 360mg/m^2 repeated every 3-4 weeks [105]. On a dailyx5 schedule, neutropenia was again dose limiting at 40-50mg/m^2/dx5, repeated every 28 days [106].

DWA2114R [(-)-(R)-2-aminomethylpyrrolidine (1,1 cyclobutanedicarboxylato)platinum(II)]

This compound (Fig. 8) shows a broader spectrum of activity in transplantable mouse tumour models than NK121, being curative in the M5076. However, it is not active against the L1210 cisplatin-resistant leukaemia, in contrast to NK121. The enantiomer(DWA2114S) showed comparable antitumour activity but was nephrotoxic in mice. Myelosuppression was dose limiting in a single phase I study of DWA2114R, the maximum tolerated dose being 800mg/m^2 [107]. When given as a 4- or 5-day continuous infusion the MTD was 1200 mg/m^2/day, gastrointestinal toxicity being dose limiting [108]. This compound is currently in phase II study in Japan.

254S [Diammine(glycolato-0,0')platinum(II)]

Unlike the other two Japanese platinum complexes just discussed, 254S (Fig. 8) contains hydroxyacetic acid, rather than 1,1-cyclobutanedicarboxylic acid as a leaving ligand. It possesses superior preclinical antitumour activity to both NK121 and DWA2114R, in being curative against the B16, M5076 and L1210 models. However, it is without activity against cisplatin acquired resistant mouse leukaemias [104]. In a phase I study of a single-dose

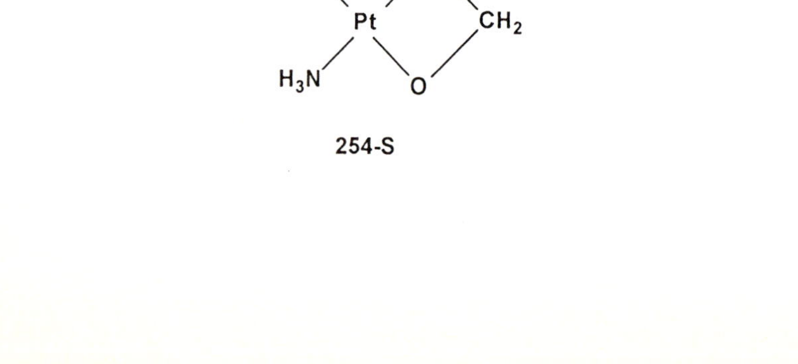

Fig. 8. Structures of NK121, DWA2114R and 254-S

schedule, thrombocytopenia was dose limiting at 120 mg/m^2, given every 4 weeks. Renal toxicity was mild and infrequent [109]. When given as a 5-day continuous infusion, dose-limiting toxicities were thrombocytopenia and leucopenia at 85 mg/m^2/120hr q 6wk [110]. In a phase II study in non-small cell lung cancer a response rate of 14% was observed [111].

Future Drug Discovery Objectives

The circumvention of clinical resistance to platinum-based chemotherapy remains a critical challenge, since there is no evidence that any of the cisplatin analogues discovered to date (some discussed here) has made an impact on this continuing problem. It seems logical that further advances must be dependent both upon an improved understanding of the underlying mechanisms involved and upon the availability of reliably predictive pre-clinical models with which to assess the therapeutic potential and selectivity of novel agents. Good progress has been made with the latter issue [56-64].

Our understanding of "classical" cellular resistance mechanisms to cisplatin is relatively well advanced, embracing impaired drug accumulation, enhanced intracellular detoxification (via the presence of elevated levels of nucleophilic molecules such as glutathione and metallothioneins), and enhanced deplatination and repair of DNA-Pt lesions [see 65-67, 112,113 for reviews]. However, our understanding of the acute response of tumour cells to platinum challenge is in its infancy, though knowledge is accruing rapidly. It is likely that future platinum-based anti-cancer drug design initiatives will need to take serious account of the molecular biological response of both normal and tumour cells to the cytotoxic insults inflicted by the present generation of platinum-based drugs.

For example, it has been shown that a 200 KDa membrane-associated glycoprotein is generated *in vitro* in mouse thymic lymphoma cells which exhibit acquired resistance to cisplatin. This protein is discretely different from the 170 KDa protein which is a primary determinant of the "multi-drug resistance" phenotype characteristic of resistance to "natural product-type" drugs such as anthracyclines, vinca alkaloids and podophyllotoxins [114]. As yet its putative role as a determinant of cisplatin resistance remains to be evaluated. Another molecule, the high-mobility group protein HMG1, can recognise DNA containing cisplatin-d(GpG) or -d(ApG) intrastrand cross-links. The significance of this protein in modulating cisplatin cytotoxicity is yet to be determined [115]. Another protein, the mitochondrial P$_1$ (hsp60), is a member of the chaperonin family of proteins and is expressed in cisplatin-resistant human ovarian carcinoma cells. Again, the role of this protein in the generation of cisplatin resistance remains to be elucidated [116].

Signal transduction pathways may also mediate cisplatin cytotoxicity; for example, activation of protein kinase C by compounds such a lyngbyatoxin A or bryostatin 1 can sensitise HeLa cells to cisplatin [117,118].

Finally, there is evidence that the expression of some genes may play a role in modulating cisplatin cytotoxicity. For example, cisplatin can initiate apoptotic cell death, presumably by interfering with bcl2 expression [119]. Others have shown that transfection of NIH3T3 cells with *ras* or c-*myc* oncogenes confers cisplatin resistance associated with impaired cellular uptake of the drug [120,121]. It may be questioned whether altered gene expression arising from transfection experiments is relevant to clinically determined cisplatin resistance. However, it should be noted that c-*fos* and c-*jun* are overexpressed in human malignant cells exposed to cisplatin, both *in vitro* and in patients, following exposure to the drug [122,123].

Clearly the mediators and modulators of platinum drug sensitivity/resistance are complex and multifocal. It is likely that new platinum-based drug discovery will need to exploit rational design based upon an improved understanding of the molecular details of platinum drug sensitivity/resistance mechanisms.

Conclusions

Cisplatin therapy has revolutionised the management in particular of patients with testicular teratoma and ovarian carcinoma, such that the former condition is now considered curative, whilst long-term remissions of advanced disease and, possibly, a low incidence of cures, is possible in the latter, although these benefits have been achieved in the face of substantial toxicities and their associated morbidity. During the (almost) 20 years which have elapsed since the introduction of cisplatin into the clinic, reliable procedures have been developed, pragmatically, to control drug-induced nephrotoxicity (hydration and diuresis) and emesis (improved application of conventional antiemetics and the discovery and development of the (more effective) $5HT_3$ antagonists). However, whilst the nephrotoxic and emetogenic sequelae of cisplatin treatment have been ameliorated by these methods, there has been no parallel reduction in other serious toxicities, notably neuropathy, hearing loss and visual impairment.

In the light of this experience, new platinum drug initiatives have been channelled primarily towards two objectives: firstly, the identification of molecules which may have a wider spectrum of clinical utility, notably to possess activity in *ab-initio* refractory and in relapsed disease; and secondly, the discovery of new drugs which retain the useful antitumour properties of cisplatin, but which are devoid of its more serious toxic limitations. The former objective has relied heavily on cisplatin (acquired) resistant mouse leukaemias for structure-activity evaluations which have identified the diaminocyclohexane ligand as a key feature for resistance circumvention.

Regrettably, mouse leukaemia models are inadequate caricatures of those human tumours which are sensitive to cisplatin and their acquired resistant counterparts predict even less faithfully for response of platinum-refractory cancers to treatment. It is perhaps not surprising therefore that compounds developed against cisplatin acquired resistant variants of mouse leukaemias fail to fulfill their preclinical promise. Moreover, the attendant toxicities may restrict the wider clinical evaluation of 1,2-diaminocyclohexane-based complexes. At present there is no evidence from any clinical study to suggest that such compounds may fulfill the clinical promise offered by their superb activities against cisplatin-refractory mouse leukaemias.

Carboplatin has been a successful example illustrating the ability to "design out" the toxic and pharmacologic limitations of the parent drug as encountered in the clinic. This drug, equiactive with its parent, has produced substantial quality-of-life benefits to patients, which may be improved upon further in the outpatient setting if clinical studies with the new orally active compound, JM216, are successful. Nonetheless, neither of these developments has targeted clinical cisplatin resistance as its major objective. The genesis of such "new generation" drugs is likely to be dependent, in large measure, upon elucidating and exploiting the complex molecular interactions, some of which have been outlined above, which may underlie the sensitivity of cisplatin-resistant tumour cells to novel platinum-containing molecules.

Acknowledgements

The work at the Institute of Cancer Research summarised herein has been supported by grants from the Cancer Research Campaign, the Medical Research Council, the Johnson Matthey Technology Centre and the Bristol Myers Squibb Company. The author is grateful to Drs Kelland and McKeage for helpful discussions and to Mrs Lesley Robertson for her skillful preparation of the manuscript.

REFERENCES

1   Rosenberg B: Platinum complexes for the treatment of cancer. Interdisciplin Sci Rev 1978 (3): 134-147
2   Harrap KR: Platinum analogues: criteria for selection. In: Muggia FM (ed) Cancer Chemotherapy 1. Martinus Nijhoff, Boston 1983 pp 171-217
3   Wolpert-De Filippes MK: Antitumor activity of cis-dichlorodiammine platinum(II). Cancer Treat Rep 1979 (63): 1453-1458
4   Guarino AM, Miller DS, Arnold ST, Pritchard JB, Davis RD, Urbanek MA, Miller TJ, Litterst CL: Platinate toxicity: Past, present and prospects. Cancer Treat Rep 1979 (63): 1475-1483
5   Harrap KR: Preclinical studies identifying carboplatin as a viable cisplatin alternative. Cancer Treat Rev 1985 (12 Suppl A):21-33
6   Schaeppi U, Heyman IA, Fleisehmann RW: Cis-dichlorodiammine platinum(II) (NSC 119875): Preclinical toxicologic evaluation of intravenous injections in dogs, monkeys and mice. Toxicol Appl Pharmacol 1973 (25): 230-241
7   Fleischman RW, Stadnicki SW, Ethier MF, Schaeppi U: Ototoxicity of cis-dichlorodiammine platinum(II) in the guinea pig. Toxicol Appl Pharmacol 1975 (33): 320 332
8   Kociba RJ, Sleight SD: Acute toxicologic and pathologic effects of cis-diamminedichloro platinum (NSC 119875) in the male rat. Cancer Chemother Rep 1971 (55): 1-8
9   Stadnicki SW, Fleischman RW, Schaeppi U, Merriam P: Cis-dichlorodiammine platinum(II) (NSC 119875): Hearing loss and other toxic effects in Rhesus monkeys. Cancer Chemother Rep 1975 (59): 467-480
10   Ward JM, Faucie KA: The nephropathology of cis-diamminedichloroplatinum(II) (NSC 119875) in male F344 rats. Toxicol Appl Pharmacol 1976 (38): 535-547
11   Madias NE, Harrington JT: Platinum nephrotoxicity. Am J Med 1978 (65): 307-314
12   Higby DJ, Wallace HJ, Jr, Albert D, Holland JF: Diamminodichloroplatinum in the chemotherapy of testicular tumors. J Urol 1974 (112): 100-104
13   Merrin CE: Treatment of genitourinary tumours with cis-dichlorodiammine platinum(II): Experience in 250 patients. Cancer Treat Rep 1979 (63): 1579-1584
14   Carter SK, Wasserman TH: The chemotherapy of urologic cancer. Cancer 1975 (36): 729-747
15   Rozencweig M, Von Hoff DD, Catane R, Muggia FM: Platinum complexes in cancer chemotherapy In: Schabel FM (ed) Antibiotics and Chemotherapy. Basel: Karger 1978 (23): 99-112
16   Williams C: Current dilemmas in the management of non-seminomatous germ cell tumors of the testis. Cancer Treat Rev 1977 (4): 275-297
17   Einhorn LH, Donohue JP: Improved chemotherapy in disseminated testicular cancer. J Urol 1977 (117): 65-69
18   Samson MK, Baker LH, Devos JM, Buroker TR, Isbicki RM, Vaitkevicius VK: Phase I clinical trial of combined therapy with vinblastine (NSC 49842), bleomycin (NSC 125066) and cis-dichlorodiammine platinum(II) (NSC 119875). Cancer Treat Rep 1976 (60): 91-97
19   Einhorn LE: Combination chemotherapy with cis-dichlorodiammine platinum(II) in disseminated testicular cancer. Cancer Treat Rep 1979 (63): 1659-1662
20   Samson MK, Stephens RL, Rivkin S, Opipari M, Maloney T, Groppe CW, Fischer R: Vinblastine, bleomycin and cis-dichlorodiammineplatinum II in disseminated testicular cancer: Preliminary report of a South West Oncology Group Study. Cancer Treat Rep 1979 (63): 1663-1667
21   Williams SD, Einhorn LH: Cisplatin chemotherapy of testicular cancer. In: Prestayko AW, Crooke ST, Carter SK (eds) Cisplatin, Current Status and New Developments. Academic Press, New York 1980 pp 323-328
22   Wiltshaw E, Kroner T: Phase II Study of cis-dichlorodiammine platinum(II) (NSC 119875) in advanced carcinoma of the ovary. Cancer Treat Rep 1976 (60): 55-60
23   Bruckner HW, Cohen CJ, Wallach RC, Kabakow B, Deppe G, Greenspan EM, Gusberg SB, Holland JF: Treatment of advanced ovarian cancer with cis-dichlorodiammineplatinum(II): Poor risk patients with intensive prior therapy. Cancer Treat Rep 1978 (62). 555-558
24   Young RC, Von Hoff DD, Gormley P, Makuch R, Cassidy J, Howser D, Bull JM: Cis-dichlorodiammineplatinum(II) for the treatment of advanced ovarian cancer. Cancer Treat Rep 1979 (63): 1539-1544
25   Wiltshaw E, Carr T: Cis-platinum(II)diamminedichloride: Clinical experience of the Royal Marsden Hospital and Institute of Cancer Research. Recent Results Cancer Res 1974 (48): 178-182
26   Merrin C: Treatment of advanced bladder cancer with cis-diamminedichloroplatinum(II) (NSC 119875): A pilot study. J Urol 1978 (119): 493-495
27   Yagoda A, Watson RC, Gonzalez-Vitale JC, Grabstaldt H, Whitmore WF: Cis-dichlorodiammineplatinum(II) in advanced bladder cancer. Cancer Treat Rep 1976 (60): 917-923
28   Herr HW: Cis-diamminedichloride platinum(II) in the treatment of advanced bladder cancer. J Urol 1980 (123): 853-855
29   Yagoda A: Cisplatin regimens in the treatment of bladder and penile cancer. In: Prestayko AW, Crooke ST, Carter SK (eds) Cisplatin, Current Status and New Developments, Academic Press, New York 1980 pp 361-374
30   Jacobs C: The role of cisplatin in the treatment of recurrent head and neck cancer. In: Prestayko AW, Crooke ST, Carter SK (eds) Cisplatin, Current Status and New Developments. New York: Academic Press 1980 pp 423-432
31   Hong WK, Bhutani E, Shapshay SM, Strong S: Induction chemotherapy of advanced previously untreated squamous cell head and neck cancer with cisplatin and bleomycin. In: Prestayko AW, Crooke ST, Carter SK (eds) Cisplatin, Current

status and New Developments. Academic Press, New York 1980, pp 431-444

32   Rozencweig M, Von Hoff DD, Slavik M, Muggia FM: Cis-diamminedichloroplatinum(II). A new anticancer drug. Ann Int Med 1977 (86): 803-812

33   Prestayko AW, D'Aoust JC, Issell BF, Crooke ST: Cisplatin (cis-diamminedichloroplatinumII). Cancer Treat Rev 1979 (6): 17-39

34   Rozencweig M, Von Hoff DD, Abele R, Muggia FM: Cisplatin. In: Pinedo JM (ed) The EORTC Cancer Chemotherapy Annual I. Exerpta Medica, Amsterdam 1980 pp 107-117

35   Randolph VL, Witles RE: Weekly administration of cis-diamminedichloroplatinum(II) without hydration or osmotic diuresis. Eur J Cancer 1978 (14): 753-756

36   Gonzalez-Vitale JC, Hayes DM, Cvitkovic E, Sternberg SS: The renal pathology in clinical trials of cis-platinum(II) diamminedichloride. Cancer 1977 (39): 1362-1371

37   Dentino M, Luft FC, Yum MN, Williams SD, Einhorn H: Long-term effect of cis-diamminedichloride platinum (CDDP) on renal function and structure in man. Cancer 1978 (41): 1274-1281

38   Hayes DM, Cvitkovic E, Golbey RB, Scheiner E, Helson L, Krakoff IH: High dose cisplatinum diamminedichloride. Cancer 1977 (39): 1372-1381

39   Krakoff IH: Nephrotoxicity of cis-dichlorodiammineplatinum(II). Cancer Treat Rep 1979 (63): 1523-1525

40   Ozols RF, Corden BJ, Collins J and Young RC: High dose cisplatin in hypertonic saline: renal effects and pharmacokinetics of a 40mg/m^2 QDx5 schedule. In: Hacker MP, Double EB, Krakoff IH (eds) Platinum Coordination Complexes in Cancer Chemotherapy. Martinus Nijhoff, Boston 1984 pp 321-329

41   Von Hoff DD, Schilsky R, Reichert CM, Reddick RL, Rozencweig M, Young RC, Muggia FM: Toxic effects of cis-dichlorodiammineplatinum(II) in man. Cancer Treat Rep 1979 (63): 1527-1532

42   Boyd MR: Status of the NCI preclinical antitumor drug discovery screen. PPO Updates 1989 (3): 1-12

43   Wolpert De Fillipes MK: Antitumour activity of cisplatin analogues. In: Prestayko AW, Crooke ST, Carter SK (eds) Cisplatin, Current Status and New Developments. Academic Press, New York 1980 pp 183-192

44   Burchenal JH, Kalaher K, Dew K, Lokys L: Rationale for the development of platinum analogs. Cancer Treat Rep 1979 (63): 1493-1498

45   Burchenal JH, Irani G, Kern K, Lokys L, Turkervich J: 1,2-Diaminocyclohexane platinum derivatives of potential clinical value. Recent Results Cancer Res 1980 (74): 146-155

46   Burchenal JH, Lokys L, Turkevich J, Ramachandran C: Rationale of combination chemotherapy. In: Prestayko AW, Crooke ST, Carter SK (eds) Cisplatin, Current Status and New Developments. Academic Press, New York 1980 pp 113-124

47   Schwartz P, Meischan SJ, Gale GR, Atkins LM, Smith AB, Walker EM Jr: Preparation and antitumour evaluation of water soluble derivatives of dichloro(1,2-diamminocyclohexane)platinum(II). Cancer Treat Rep 1977 (61): 1519-1525

48   Kidani Y, Noji M, Tashiro T: Antitumour activity of platinum (II) complexes of 1,2-diaminocyclohexane isomers. Gann 1980 (71): 637-643

49   Kidani Y, Inagaki K, Iigo M, Hoshi A, Kazuo K: Antitumour activity of 1,2-diaminocyclohexane-platinum complexes against sarcoma-180 ascites form. J Med Chem 1978 (21 part 12): 1315-1318

50   Mathé G, Kidani Y, Noji M, Maral R, Borut C, Chenu E: Antitumour activity of I-OHP in mice. Cancer Lett. 1985 (27): 135-143

51   Sekiguchi M, Eriguchi M, Shiroko Y, Akiyama N, Mikamo S: Chemosensitivity screening *in vitro* of various cultured human cancer cell lines to a new platinum complex. I-OHP: Oxalato (trans I-1,2-diaminocyclohexane)platinum(II). Annals Oncol 1992 (3 Suppl 1): Abs 194

52   Anderson WK, Quagliato DA, Haugwitz RD, Narayanan VL and Wolpert-De Fillipes MK: Synthesis, physical properties and antitumour activity of tetraplatin and related tetrachloroplatinum(IV) stereoisomers of 1,2-diaminocyclohexane. Cancer Treat Rep 1986 (70): 997-1002

53   Gibbons GR, Wyrick S, Chaney SG: Rapid reduction of tetrachloro(D,L-*trans*) 1,2-diaminocyclohexaneplatinum(IV) (Tetraplatin) in RPMI tissue culture medium. Cancer Res 1989 (49): 1402-1407

54   Carfagna PF, Poma A, Wyrick SD, Holbrook DJ, Chaney SG: Comparisons of tetrachloro (D,L-*trans*) 1,2-diaminocyclohexaneplatinum(IV) biotransformations in the plasma of Fisher 344 rats at therapeutic and toxic doses. Cancer Chemother Pharmacol 1991 (27): 335-341

55   Rose WC, Schurig JE, Bradner WT, Huftalen JB: Antitumour activity and toxicity of cis-diamminedichloroplatinum (II) analogs. Cancer Treat Rep 1982 (66): 135-146

56   Goddard PM, Valenti MR, Harrap KR: The role of murine tumour models and their acquired platinum-resistant counterparts in the evaluation of novel platinum antitumour agents: a cautionary note. Ann Oncol 1991 (2): 535-540

57   Hills CA, Kelland G, Abel G, Siracky J, Wilson AP, Harrap KR: Biological properties of ten human ovarian carcinoma cell lines: calibration in vitro against four platinum complexes. Br. J. Cancer 1989 (59): 527-534

58   Harrap KR, Jones M, Siracky J, Pollard LA, Kelland LR: The establishment, characterization and calibration of human ovarian carcinoma xenografts for the evaluation of novel platinum anticancer drugs. Ann Oncol 1990 (1): 65-76

59   Kelland LR, Jones M, Abel G, Valenti M, Gwynne J, Harrap KR: Human ovarian carcinoma cell lines and companion xenografts: a disease-oriented approach to new platinum anticancer drug discovery. Cancer Chemother Pharmacol 1992 (30): 43-50

60   Kelland LA, Murrer BA, Abel G, Harrap KR: Structure-activity relationships in a series of novel platinum(II) and platinum(IV) ammine/amine complexes evaluated against a panel of human

ovarian carcinoma cell lines. J Cell Pharmacol 1991 (2): 331-342

61 Giandomenico CM, Abrams MJ, Murrer BA, Vollano JF, Harrap KR, Kelland LR, Morgan SE: Synthesis and reactions of a new class of orally active Pt(IV) antitumour complexes. In: Howell SB (ed) Platinum and Other Metal Coordination Complexes in Cancer Chemotherapy. Plenum Press, New York 1991 pp 93-100

62 Harrap KR, Murrer BA, Giandomenico C, Morgan SA, Kelland LR, Jones M, Goddard PM and Schurig J: Ammine/amine platinum(IV) dicarboxylates: a novel class of complexes which circumvent intrinsic cisplatin resistance. In: Howell SB (ed) Platinum and Other Metal Coordination Complexes in Cancer Chemotherapy. Plenum Press, New York 1991 pp 391-399

63 Harrap KR, Kelland LR, Jones M, Goddard PM, Orr RM, Morgan SE, Murrer BA, Abrams MJ, and Giandomenico CM: Platinum coordination complexes which circumvent cisplatin resistance. Adv Enzyme Regulation 1991 (31): 31-43

64 McKeage MJ, Morgan SE, Boxall FE, Hard GC, Murrer B, Judson I, Harrap KR: Acute toxicology of orally administered *bis*-acetato-ammine dichloro(cyclohexylamine)platinum(IV) (JM216) in rodents. Proc Amer Assoc Cancer Res 1992 (33) Abs 3197

65 De Graeff A, Slebos RJC, Rodenhuis S: Resistance to cisplatin and analogues: mechanisms and potential clinical implications. Cancer Chemother Pharmacol 1988 (22): 325-332

66 Andrews PA, Howell SB: Cellular pharmacology of cisplatin: perspectives on mechanisms of acquired resistance. Cancer Cells (Cold Spring Harbor) 1990 (2): 35-43

67 McKeage MJ, Higgins JD (III), Kelland LR: Platinum and other metal coordination compounds in cancer chemotherapy. Br J Cancer 1991 (64): 788-792

68 Kelland LR, Murrer BA, Abel G, Giandomenico CM, Mistry P, Harrap KR: Ammine/amine platinum (IV) dicarboxylates: a novel class of platinum complex exhibiting selective cytotoxicity to intrinsically cisplatin-resistant human ovarian cell lines. Cancer Res 1992 (52): 822-828

69 Kelland LR, Mistry P, Abel G, Loh SY, O'Neill CF, Murrer BA, Harrap KR: Mechanism-related circumvention of *cis*-diamminedichloroplatinum(II) resistance using two pairs of human ovarian carcinoma cell lines by ammine/amine platinum(IV) dicarboxylates. Cancer Res 1992 (52): 3857-3864

70 Knox RJ, Friedlos F, Lydall DA, Roberts JJ: Mechanism of cytotoxicity of anticancer platinum drugs: Evidence that *cis*-diamminedichloro-platinum(II) and *cis*-diammine (1,1-cyclobutane-dicarboxylato)platinum(II) differ only in the kinetics of their interaction with DNA. Cancer Res 1986 (46): 1972-1979

71 Farrell N, Qu Y, Hacker MP: Cytotoxicity and antitumor activity of bis(platinum) complexes. A novel class of platinum complexes active in cell lines resistant to both cisplatin and 1,2-diaminocyclohexane complexes. J Med Chem 1990 (33): 2179-2184

72 Farrell N, Qu Y, Feng L, Van Houten B: Comparison of chemical reactivity, cytotoxicity, interstrand cross linking and DNA sequence specificity of bis(platinum) complexes containing monodentate of bidentate coordination spheres with their monomeric analogues. Biochem 1990 (29) 9522-9531

73 Van Beusichem M, Farrell N: Activation of the trans geometry in platinum antitumor complexes. Synthesis, characterisation and biological activity of complexes with the planar ligands pyridine, N-methylimidazole, thiazole and quinoline. Crystal and molecular structure of *trans*-dichlorobis(thiazole)platinum(II). Inog Chem 1992 (31) 634-639

74 Farrell N, Kelland LR, Roberts JD, Van Beusichem M: Activation of the trans geometry in platinum antitumor complexes: A survey of the cytotoxicity of trans complexes containing planar ligands in murine L1210 and human tumor panels and studies on their mechanism of action. Cancer Res 1992 (52): 5065-5072

75 Hill JM, Loeb E, Pardue A, Khan A, King JJ, Akman C, Hill NO: Platinum analogs of clinical interest. Cancer Treat Rep 1979 (63): 1509-1513

76 Ribaud P, Alcock N, Burchenal JH, Young C, Muggia F, Mathe G: Preclinical trial in a phase I-II trial and pharmacokinetics in man of malonato-platinum (MP) Proc Am Soc Clin Oncol 1979 (20): 336

77 Ribaud P, Kelsen DP, Alcock N, Garcia-Giralt E, Dulbouch P, Young CC, Muggia FM, Burchenal JH, Mathe G: Preclinical and phase I studies of malonatoplatinum. Recent Results Cancer Res 1980 (74): 156-162

78 Kelsen DP, Scher H, Alcock N et al: Phase I clinical trial and pharmacokinetics of 4'carboxy-phthalato(1,2-diaminocyclohexane) platinum(II). Cancer Res 1982 (42): 4831-4835

79 Kelsen DP, Scher H, Burchenal J: Phase I and early phase II trials of 4'carboxyphthalato (1,2-diaminocyclohexane) platinum II. In: Hacker MP, Double EB, Krakoff IH (eds) Platinum Coordination Complexes in Cancer Chemotherapy. Martinus Nijhoff, Boston 1984 pp 310-320

80 Christian MC, Kohn E, Sarosy G, Link C, Davis P, Adams D, Weiss RB, Brewster L, Lombardo F, Reed E: Phase I and pharmacologic study of ormaplatin (OP)/tetraplatin. Proc Amer Soc Clin Oncol 1992 (11): Abs 291

81 Tutsch KD, Arzoomanian RZ, Alberti D, Feierabend C, Robins HI, Spriggs DR: Phase I and pharmacokinetic study of ormaplatin. Proc Amer Assoc Cancer Res 1992 (33): Abs 3202

82 Schilder RJ, La Creta FP, Pereg RP, Nash S, Hamilton TC, Goldstein LJ, Young RC, Ozols RF, O'Dwyer PJ: Phase I/pharmacokinetic study of ormaplatin (tetraplatin, NSC 363812). Proc Amer Assoc Cancer Res 1992 (33): Abs 3211

83 O'Rourke T, Rodriguez G, Eckardt J, Kuhn J, Burris H, Hardy J, Weiss G, Von Hoff D: Phase I clinical trial of ormaplatin (NSC 363812) given on a dailyx5 every 28 day schedule. Proc Amer Assoc Cancer Res 1992 (33): Abs 3215

84   Trump DL, Petros W, Chaney S, Smith DC, Fangmeier J, Brown TD, Goldberg H: Phase I clinical trial and study of the pharmacokinetics and metabolism of ormaplatin (tetraplatin, NSC 363812). Proc Amer Assoc Cancer Res 1992 (33): Abs 3217

85   Extra JM, Espie M, Calvo F, Ferme C, Mignot L, Marty M: Phase I study of oxaliplatin in patients with advanced cancer. Cancer Chemother Pharmacol 1990 (25): 299-303

86   Caussanel JP, Levi F, Brienza S, Misset JL, Itzhaki M, Adam R, Milano G, Hecquet B, Mathé G: Phase I trial of 5 day continuous venous infusion of oxaliplatin at circadian rhythm - modulated rate compared with constant rate. JNCI 1990 (82): 1046-1050

87   Vermorken JB, ten Bokkel Huinink WW, McVie JG, van der Vijgh WJF, Pinedo HM: Clinical experience with 1, 1-diaminomethylcyclohexane (sulphato) platinum(II) (TNO6). In: Hacker MP, Douple EB, Krakoff IJ (eds) Platinum Coordination Complexes in Cancer Chemotherapy. Martinus Nijhoff, Boston 1984 pp 330-343

88   Wagstaff AJ, Ward A, Benfield P, Heel RC: Carboplatin: A preliminary review of its pharmacodynamic and pharmacokinetic properties and therapeutic efficacy in the treatment of cancer. Drugs 1989 (37-2): 163-186

89   Yarbo JW (ed): Carboplatin (JM8) update: Current perspectives and future directions. Sem Oncol 1992 (19 Suppl 2): 1-164

90   Mangioni C, Bolis G, Pecorelli S, Bragman K, Epis A, Favalli G, Gambino A, Landoni F, Presti M, Torri W, Vassena L, Zanaboni F, and Marsoni S: Randomised trial in ovarian cancer comparing cisplatin and carboplatin. JNCI 1989 (81): 1464-1468

91   Advanced Ovarian Cancer Trialists Group: Chemotherapy in advanced ovarian cancer: an overview of randomised clinical trials. Br Med J 1991 (303) 884-893

92   Gore M, Fryatt I, Wiltshaw E, Dawson T, Robinson B and Clavert A: Cisplatin/carboplatin cross-resistance in ovarian cancer. Br J Cancer 1989 (60) 767-769

93   Eisenhauer E, Swerton K, Sturgeon J, Fine S, O'Reilly S, Canetta R: Carboplatin therapy for recurrent ovarian carcinoma: National Cancer Institute of Canada experience and a review of the literature. In: Bunn P, Canetta R, Ozols R and Rozencweig M (eds) Carboplatin; Current Perspectives and Future Directions. WB Saunders Company, Philadelphia 1990 pp 133-140

94   Trask C, Silverstone A, Ash CM, Earl H, Irwin C, Bakker A, Tobias JS, Souhami RL: A randomized trial of carboplatin versus iproplatin in untreated ovarian cancer. J Clin Oncol 1991 (9): 1131-1137

95   Bitha P, Carvajal SG, Citarella RV, Delos Santos EF, Durr FE, Hlavka JJ, Lang SA, Lindsay HL, Thomas JP, Wallace RE, Lin Y: Water soluble third generation antitumour platinum complexes, [2,2-bis (aminomethyl)-1, 3-propanediol-N, N'] [1,1-cyclobutanedicarboxylato(2-)-O,O'] platinum(II) and [1,1-cyclobutanedicarboxylato(2-)-O,O']

[tetrahydro-4H-pyran-4, 4-dimethanamine-N,N']. J Med Chem 1989 (32(8)): 2015-2020

96   Meijer C, Mulder NH, Timmer-Bosscha H, Meersma GJ, De Vries EG: Role of GSH in the efficacy of 7 platinum(Pt) compounds in 2 cisplatin(CDDP)-resistant human cell lines. Proc Amer Assoc Cancer Res 1991 (32): Abs 2427

97   Dodion PF, de Valeriola D, Crepeigne N, Kantrowitz JD, Piccart M, Wery F, Kergier J, Egorin MJ, Forrest A, Bachur NR, Alaerts P, Carver A, Rastogi R, Hammershaimb L, Saletan S: Phase I clinical and pharmacokinetic study of zeniplatin, a new platinum complex. Annals Oncol 1991 (2): 589-596

98   Jones AL, Mckeage M, Davies C, Holburn J, Ashley SE, Rastogi R, Townsend H, Smith IE: Phase II study of zeniplatin in advanced non small cell lung cancer. Cancer Chemother Pharmacol 1992 (in press)

99   Aamdal S, Piccart M, Wanders J, Rastogi RB, Schwartsman G, Franklin HR, Kaye SB: Phase (II) study of zeniplatin/CL 286,558) [2,2-bis(aminomethyl)-1,3 propanediol-N,N'] [1,1-cyclobutanedicarboxylato(2-)O,O'] platinum(II) in patients with advanced melanoma. *Poster presented at the Sixth International Symposium on platinum and other metal coordination compounds (San Diego, Ca) Jan (23-26) 1991, but not published in the conference proceedings*

100   Olver I, Green M, Peters W, Zimet A, Toner G, Bishop J, Ketelbey W, Astogi R, Birkhofer M: A pilot phase (II) study of zeniplatin in metastatic melanoma. Annals Oncol 1992 (3 Suppl 1): Abs 345

101   Piccart M, Kerger J, Tueni E, van der Schueren E, Kennes C, Bartholomeus S, Vantongelen K, Rastogi R, Birkhofer M: Phase II trial of zeniplatin (CL 286, 558; ZNP) as second line treatment in metastatic breast cancer (MBC). Proc Amer Assoc Cancer Res 1991 (32): Abs 1222

102   Willemse PH, Giettera JA, Sleijfer DT, Mulder NH, de Vries EG, de Halleux F, Rastogi RB, Birkhofer M: Activity of a third generation platinum compound zeniplatin (CL 286, 558) in patients with recurrent ovarian cancer. Proc Amer Soc Clin Oncol 1991 (10): Abs 626

103   Ceulemans F, Duprez P, Vindevogel A, Tueni E, Piccart M, Kerger J, Rastogi R, de Halleux F: Enloplatin (CL287, 110): Phase I study in patients with advanced solid tumours. *Poster presented at the Sixth International Symposium on platinum and other metal coordination compounds (San Diego, Ca) Jan (23-26) 1991, but not published in the conference proceedings*

104   Majima H: Clinical studies with cisplatin analogues, 254-S, DWA 2114R and NK121. In: Howell SB (ed) Platinum and Other Metal Coordination Compounds in Cancer Chemotherapy. Plenum Press, New York 1991 pp 345-355

105   Fukuoka M, Niitani H, Hasegawa K, Majima H, Hino M, Furue H, Tsukagoshi S, Fujita H, Ohta K, Furuse K, Kimura I, Katoh T: Phase I study of a new platinum compound, NK121. Proc Amer Soc Clin Oncol 1989 (8): Abs 240

106   Hughes GR, O'Dwyer PJ, Walczak J, La Creta FP, Cohen I, Kowal C, Boyd RA, Whitfield LR: Phase I/pharmacokinetic study of the new platinum

compound CI-973 on a 5-day schedule. Proc Amer Assoc Cancer Res 1991 (32): Abs 1190

107 Ariyoshi Y, Ota K: Preclinical and clinical evaluation of toxicities and antitumour activities of cisplatin analogues. Jpn J Cancer Chemother 1989 (16): 1379-1385

108 Tamura K, Makino S, Araki Y: A phase I study of a new cisplatin derivative for haematological malignancies. Cancer 1990 (66): 2059-2063

109 Ariyoshi Y, Ota K, Wakui A, Majima H, Niitani H, Ogawa M, Imuyama Y, Yoshida O, Taguchi T, Kimura I, Kato T: Phase I study of [glycolato-O,O'] diammine platinum(II) (254-5). Proc Amer Soc Clin Oncol 1988 (7): Abs 222.

110 Sasaki Y, Amano T, Morita M, Shinkai T, Eguchi K, Tamura T, Ohe Y, Kojima A, Saijo N: Phase I study and pharmacological analysis of cis-diammine(glycolato)platinum(II) (254-5; NSC 375101d) administered by 5-day continuous intravenous infusion. Cancer Res 1991 (51): 1472-1477

111 Fukuda M, Shinkai T, Eguchi K, Sasaki Y, Tamura T, Ohe Y, Kojima A, Oshita F, Hara K, Saijo N: Phase II study of (glycolate-O,O') diammine-platinum(II), a novel platinum complex in the treatment of non-small cell lung cancer. Cancer Chemother Pharmacol 1990 (26): 393-396

112 Kelley SL, Rozencweig M: Resistance to platinum compounds: mechanisms and beyond. Eur J Cancer Clin Oncol 1989 (25): 1135-1140

113 Scanlon KJ, Kashani-Sabet M, Tone T, Funato T. Cisplatin resistance in human cancers. Pharmac Ther 1991 (52): 385-406

114 Kuwai K, Kumatani N, Georges E, Ling V: Identification of a membrane glycoprotein overexpressed in murine lymphoma sublines resistant to cis-diamminodichloroplatinum(II). J Biol Chem 1990 (265) 13137-13142

115 Pil PM, Lippard SJ: Specific binding of chromosomal protein HMG1 to DNA damaged by the anticancer drug cisplatin. Science 1992 (256): 234-237

116 Enns RE and Howell SB: Isolation of a gene associated with resistance to cisplatin. In: Howell SB (ed) Platinum and Other Metal Coordination Compounds in Cancer Chemotherapy. Plenum Press, New York 1991 pp 213-219

117 Basu A, Kozikowski AP, Sato K, Lazo JS: Cellular sensitisation to cis-diamminodichloro platinum (II) by novel analogues of the protein kinase C activator lyngbyatoxin A. Cancer Res 1991 (51): 2511-2514

118 Basu A, Lazo JS: Sensitization of human cervical carcinoma cells to cis-diamminedichloroplat-inum(II) by bryostatin 1. Cancer Res 1991 (52): 3119-3124

119 Eastman A: Activation of programmed cell death by anticancer agents: cisplatin as a model system. Cancer Cells 1990 (2): 275-280

120 Isonishi S, Hom DK, Thiebaut FB, Mann SC, Andrews PA, Basu A, Lazo JS, Eastman A, Howell SB: Expression of the C-Ha-ras oncogene in mouse NIH3T3 cells induces resistance to cisplatin. Cancer Res 1991 (51): 5903-5909

121 Niimi S, Nakagawa K, Yokata J, Tsunokawa Y, Nishio K, Terashima Y, Shibuya M, Terada M, Saijo N: Resistance to anticancer drugs in NIH 3T3 cells transfected with c-myc and/or c-Ha-ras oncogenes. Br J Cancer 1991 (63): 237-241

122 Scanlon KJ, Jiao L, Funato T, Wang W, Tone T, Rossi JJ, Kashani-Sabet M: Ribozyme-mediated cleavage of c-fos mRNA reduces gene expression of DNA synthesis enzymes and metallothionein. Proc Natl Acad Sci (USA) 1991 (88): 10591-10595

123 Rubin E, Kharbanda S, Gunji H, Weichselbaum R, Kufe D: Cis-diamminedichloro platinum(II) induces c-jun expression in human myeloid leukaemia cells: potential involvement of a protein kinase C-dependent signalling pathway. Cancer Res 1992 (52): 878-882

Pharmacological Intervention with Signal Transduction

Garth Powis

Arizona Cancer Center, University of Arizona Health Sciences Center, Tucson, AZ 85725, U.S.A.

The Need for New Types of Anticancer Drugs

It has been 50 years since the first anticancer drug of the modern era, nitrogen mustard, underwent clinical trial in a cancer patient [1]. Nitrogen mustard was introduced into general clinical practice in 1949. Since that time there has been a steady increase in the number of anticancer drugs so that in the U.S.A. there are now 45 officially approved anticancer drugs excluding steroidal agents and radiopharmaceuticals [2]. Despite this large number of drugs the early hope that chemotherapy would provide a major check against cancer has not been realised. Today, chemotherapy is curative for about 12% of human cancers, including choriocarcinoma, acute lymphocytic leukaemia, Hodgkin's disease and testicular cancer. However, most human cancers, those causing over 75% of cancer deaths including lung, colon, breast and prostate cancer, are refractory to chemotherapy. Survival rates for cancer patients in the U.S.A. are about 50%, compared to 40% in the early 1960s, before the widespread use of chemotherapy [3]. There is clearly a need for new treatments and approaches to dealing with cancer and this includes new types of cancer drugs.

Most of the anticancer drugs in use today have been developed by the random screening in animal tumour models of large numbers of chemical compound or natural product extracts. There are just a few cases of rationally developed anticancer drugs, 5-fluorouracil being an example [4]. Currently available anticancer drugs act mostly by preventing the synthesis of DNA or by interfering with DNA function. This is probably because the animal models by which these drugs were discovered were based on inhibiting the growth of rapidly growing, transplantable leukaemias in mice, which appears to select for DNA-active drugs [5]. With so little known about the underlying biological difference between the cancer cell and a normal cell, there was also an intellectual bias towards developing DNA-active drugs, because the rate of DNA synthesis was an obvious biochemical difference between a cancer cell and a normal cell. We now know that there is little wrong with DNA synthesis in a cancer cell - it is just out of control. The analogy can be made to a car speeding down the highway. A wrench in the engine will stop the car, but it will also stop slower moving cars. It makes more sense to target the driver who is making the car go too fast, than to try to halt every car completely. Through the recent advances in the knowledge of the molecular and cellular biology of the cancer cell we are in a position to try to remedy the faulty control mechanisms that make the cancer cell grow out of control.

Cancer as a Disease of Intracellular Signalling

The underlying biological difference between a cancer cell and a normal cell is the presence in the cancer cell of mutated or overexpressed developmental genes, called oncogenes, together with the loss of tumour suppressor genes [6,7]. The combination of more than one oncogene and the loss of tumour suppressor genes leads to the malignant transformation of a cell [8]. The major, if not the only function, of oncogenes appears to be to code for proteins that are components of intracellular signalling pathways. This includes nuclear oncogenes that encode transcription regulatory factors [9]. An important action of the signalling pathways is to transmit the messages generated by the interaction of growth factors with their receptors on the cell surface, to specific sets of genes in the nucleus that determine the cellular response to the growth factor. Oncogenes can lead to the constitutive activation of some of these intracellular signalling pathways. Thus, cancer can reasonably be considered a disease of intracellular signalling.

Targeting Anticancer Drugs Against Intracellular Signalling Pathways

The intracellular signalling pathways that mediate the effects of oncogenes on cell transformation present attractive target sites for pharmacological intervention. Even if the oncoprotein itself is not amenable to selective inhibition by a small molecule drug, there are many other sites along the signalling pathways that can be modulated by drugs. This is a relatively new approach to developing anticancer drugs and we do not yet know if it will produce a major therapeutic benefit in humans. There are, as yet, no anticancer drugs in clinical use that have been specifically developed as inhibitors of intracellular signalling. However, this situation is likely to change in the near future. The purpose of this review is to consider some of the potential problems to developing this type of anticancer drug. Some inhibitors of intracellular signalling pathways that are candidates for clinical development will be discussed, and the signalling inhibitory properties of some currently used anticancer drugs will be reviewed.

Degeneracy of Intracellular Signalling as an Aid to Drug Development

Many of the intracellular signalling pathways that are activated by oncogenes are used by cells for normal growth and metabolic functions. This naturally raises the question of the specificity of any drug that inhibits intracellular signalling for the cancer cell compared to a normal cell. There is considerable redundancy to growth factor signalling and the degeneracy of intracellular signalling pathways may aid our efforts at selective anticancer drug development. More than one growth factor is required for the proliferation of a normal cell so that during regulated cell growth multiple signalling pathways are activated. Furthermore, one growth factor can activate many signalling pathways [10,11]. An example of signalling degeneracy *in vivo* is found in mice engineered to lack the c-*src* proto-oncogene [12]. The c-*src* protein tyrosine kinase is highly conserved across species, suggesting it might be involved in an essential cellular function. Despite this, mice lacking c-*src* grow relatively normally with the only abnormality being osteoporosis. The apparent explanation is that other genes coding for related protein tyrosine kinases, such as *yes* and *fyn*, take over the role of c-*src* in the deficient mice. Since an oncogene may activate just one of many signalling pathways, it should be possible to use a drug to inhibit the oncogene-activated pathway without also affecting the other signalling pathways necessary for normal cell growth and metabolism. The concept is illustrated in Figure 1. A caveat to this concept is that if several signalling pathways have to be inhibited in a cancer cell in order to reverse malignant transformation, there may not be enough redundancy among the signalling pathways to save the normal cell. Recent evidence suggests there may be signalling pathways specifically associated with cell growth and transformation [11,13], so that it might be possible to develop drugs to selectively inhibit these pathways without affecting signalling pathways necessary for normal cell function, for example hormone and neurotransmitter action.

The Oncogene, a Switch or a Continuous Event?

An important question is whether oncogene expression is a switch or a continuous event necessary for malignant transformation. An oncogene could act as a single-time event (a switch) that allows a cell to proceed from a

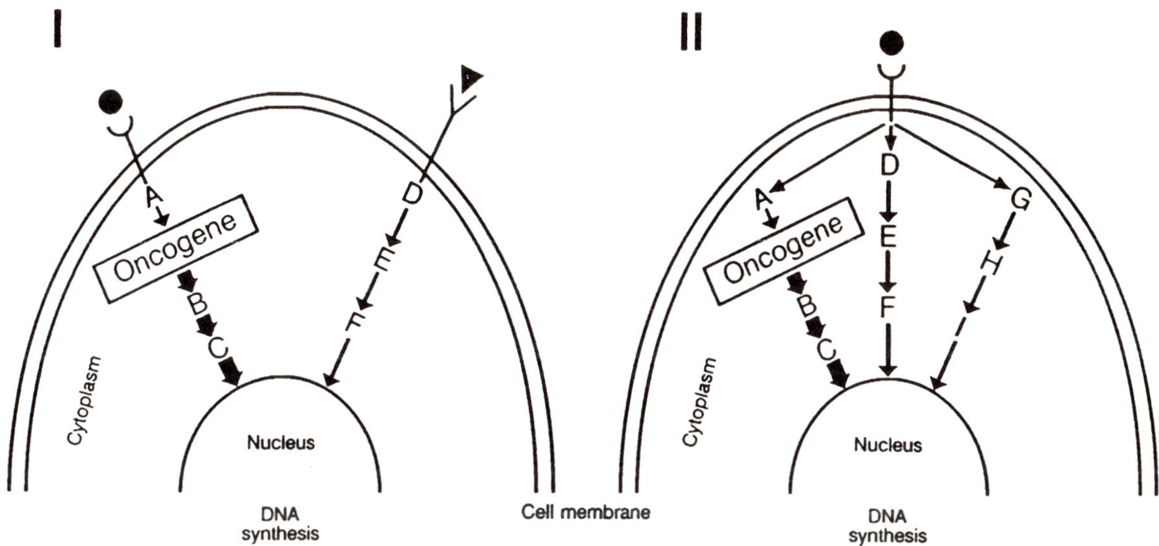

Fig. 1. Degeneracy of growth factor signalling.
I: Different growth factors activate their own signalling pathways, each of which can independently stimulate cell growth. II: A growth factor activates multiple signalling pathways and each pathway can independently stimulate cell growth. In both cases an oncogene is shown activating just one of the signalling pathways (a dark arrow). A drug that inhibits the oncogene-activated pathway could, thus, leave the alternate signalling pathways unaffected.

non-transformed to a transformed state, for example by giving a partly transformed cell a growth advantage over surrounding normal cells, thus allowing its clonal expansion. In this case, attempts to treat the cell with a drug that inhibits the oncogene will be too late, since the oncogene is no longer necessary for the maintenance of the malignant state. Evidence that this is not the case comes from the extensively studied oncogene *ras*. Inhibition of oncogenic *ras* in experimentally transformed cells through the use of antibodies [14], antisense oligonucleotides [15] or ribozymes [16] clearly shows that transformation can be reversed by inhibiting this single oncogene. That is, *ras* expression appears to be a necessary continuous event for transformation. On the other hand, it cannot be assumed that, because an oncogene is found in a tumour cell, it is essential for the maintenance of the transformed state. Studies of melanoma cells from different metastatic deposits in the same patient have shown a heterogeneous distribution of oncogenic *ras* [17]. Since the tumour is presumably clonal in origin, in this case *ras* cannot be essential for the initiation or maintenance of all of the different tumour deposits.

Will More than One Signalling Drug Be Necessary to Inhibit Cancer Cell Growth?

Tumorigenesis is a multistep process requiring the activation of more than one oncogene and the loss of tumour suppressor genes [18]. While a drug active against a single oncogene may be sufficient to return a transformed cell to a pretransformed state, the cell will likely still be abnormal because it has other expressed oncogenes. It might be better, or even necessary, to inhibit several oncogenes to return the cell to a stable, non-transformed state. Even though a drug may be active against an experimentally transformed cell, derived by the expression of an oncogene in an already immortalised cell line, we do not know whether it will be active by itself against a spontaneously arising human cancer. For activity to be seen, it might have to be combined with drugs that inhibit the other oncogenes in the tumour. We have little experience of developing anticancer drugs that do not have single-agent activity that may have to be combined with other single agent-inactive drugs. Developing such agents clinically would present a considerable departure from the way anticancer drugs are currently developed.

Drug Resistance

A major cause for the failure of current cancer chemotherapy is drug resistance [19]. Intrinsic resistance is the mechanism by which a cancer cell fails to respond to a cancer drug to which some other cells respond. It implies that the problem somehow lies with the cancer cell, not with an ineffective drug. Since most anticancer drugs are inactive against most cancer cells, it is convenient but somewhat meaningless to place the blame on the cancer cell. The solution to the problem is more effective anticancer drugs. Some tumours will initially respond to an anticancer drug but in subsequent courses of treatment lose this response. This acquired drug resistance, on the other hand, will likely remain a problem even for newer types of anticancer drugs. Presumably, acquired drug resistance would be less of a problem if we had effective drugs that could kill cancer cells on their first application. However, experience with antibacterial drugs shows that even with highly effective drugs resistance can develop among a population of rapidly dividing cells. Even if a cell develops resistance this will be of little consequence unless the resistant cell population can be expanded. The frequency of the development of resistance is related in part to the growth rate of the affected cell population. With anticancer drugs the rate at which resistance develops would be expected to be considerably lower than with bacterial cells. We do not yet know if resistance can develop to antisignalling drugs. However, *a priori* there is no reason to think it would not and indeed it would be surprising, given the known genetic instability of cancer cells, if resistance did not develop. A traditional way of preventing the development of resistance among bacterial cells is to use high-dose combination chemotherapy from the start of treatment. This is probably the way that antisignalling drugs will have to be given.

Cytostatic or Cytotoxic?

Drugs that reverse the effect of an oncogene would be expected to have cytostatic rather than cytotoxic effects on a cancer cell. In fact, the term cytotoxic as commonly used to refer to cell destruction is inappropriate, and the term cytolytic more correctly refers to the destruction of a cell. Thus, even though a tumour cell might be returned to a non-transformed state where, presumably, it would be subjected to the usual physiological controls on growth, it will continue to be a potential threat to the host should the inhibitory effects of the drug be removed. This could occur if the drug treatment is terminated, or if resistance to the drug develops. However, even a cytostatic drug will cause a reduction in tumour mass (regression). The size of a tumour is determined by a balance between new cell production and the loss of cells due to necrosis and apoptosis [20]. Thus, if new cell production is halted, the mass of a tumour will decrease. This is illustrated with anticancer drugs that act as antimetabolites, which would also be expected to be cytostatic but not cytolytic, and where tumour regression can be seen. It may be that once cancer cell proliferation has been halted the body can begin to eliminate the cancer cells by an immune mechanism [21].

Growth Factor Signalling Pathways

Before discussing some of the potential target sites and strategies for developing antisignalling drugs it is necessary to briefly review some of the signalling pathways activated by growth factors. Two major pathways are shown in Figure 2. In the first pathway a mitogenic peptide such as bombesin acts on a 7-pass membrane spanning receptor coupled to a specific guanine nucleotide binding (G) protein of the Gq class, to activate a membrane-bound phosphatidylinositol phospholipase C (PtdInsPLC), PtdInsPLC-ß [22]. There are at least 14 forms of PtdInsPLCs and 4 major classes (PtdInsPLC-α, ß, γ, and δ) so far identified. PtdInsPLC hydrolyses a minor membrane phospholipid, phosphatidylinositol(4,5)bisphosphate (PtdIns(4,5)P_2), to give the water soluble inositol(1,4,5)trisphosphate (Ins(1,4,5)P_3) and a lipophilic diacylglycerol (DAG) [23]. Ins(1,4,5)P_3 releases Ca^{2+} from non-mitochondrial stores producing a transient increase in the cytoplasmic free Ca^{2+} concentration ([Ca^{2+}] while diacylglycerol is an activator of a Ca^{2+} and phospholipid-dependent

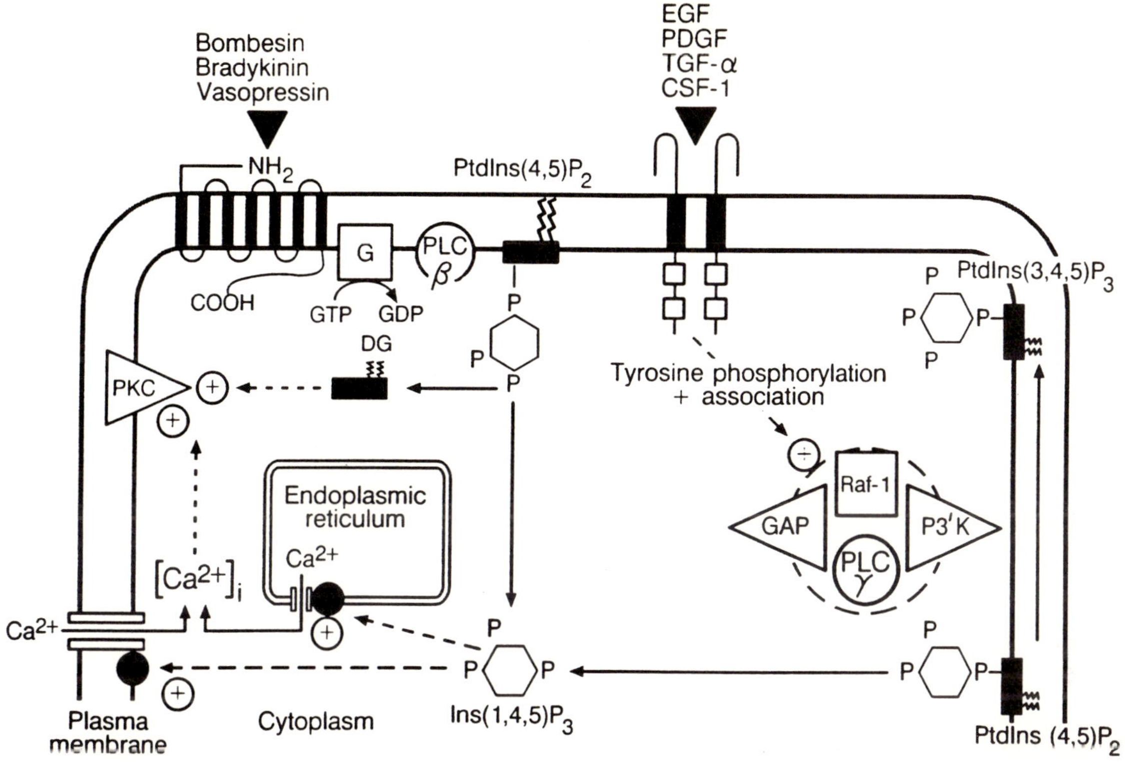

Fig. 2. Growth factor signalling pathways

protein serine/threonine kinase, protein kinase C (PKC) [24]. Proteins phosphorylated by PKC include growth factor receptors, nuclear transcription factors as well as PtdInsPLC-ß itself, which decreases the affinity for its regulatory G protein. Together, the increase in $[Ca^{2+}]$ and the increased activity of protein kinase C leads to a sequence of events that culminate in DNA synthesis and cell proliferation. Other inositol phosphates in addition to $Ins(1,4,5)P_3$ are formed in the cell [23,25]. Phosphorylation of $Ins(1,4,5)P_3$ by a specific 3-kinase gives inositol(1,3,4,5)-terakisphosphate($Ins(1,3,4,5)P_4$), which may act to refill intracellular Ca^{2+} stores and could function together with $Ins(1,4,5)P_3$ in the activation of Ca^{2+}-mediated responses [26].

In the second pathway the binding of a growth factor such as platelet-derived growth factor (PDGF) to its plasma membrane receptor causes the receptor monomers to dimerise and then to phosphorylate each other on tyrosine residues [27]. This permits a conformational change in the receptor that enhances its protein tyrosine kinase activity toward other sub-strates [28]. It also provides phosphotyrosine binding sites on the receptor for the recruitment of specific cytoplasmic enzymes that contain a src-homology-2 (SH2) domain that binds with high affinity to certain phosphotyrosines [29]. Thus, some cytoplasmic enzymes are brought into close proximity with their substrates located at the plasma membrane. One such enzyme is PtdInsPLC-γ, which is also phosphorylated on tyrosine by the ligand-activated PDGF receptor [30]. Both recruitment and tyrosine phosphorylation may account for why ligand activation of protein tyrosine kinase growth factor receptors, such as the PDGF receptor or epidermal growth factor (EGF) receptor, leads to an increase in the hydrolysis of PtdIns $(4,5)P_2$ and an elevation of $[Ca^{2+}]_{i-}$. Another cytoplasmic enzyme that is tyrosine phosphorylated by protein tyrosine kinases is phosphatidylinositol-3-kinase (PtdIns-3-kinase) [31,32]. This enzyme phosphorylates PtdIns, including PtdIns(4,5)P2, on the 3 position of the myo-inositol ring to give a class of PtdIns that are not substrates for hydrolysis by PtdInsPLC [33]. In addition to being tyrosine phosphorylated by the PDGF-receptor, PtdIns -3-kinase associates with the receptor through SH2 domain binding. The mechanism by which PtdIns-3-phosphates stimulate cell proliferation is not yet known but that may be involved in cytoskeleton reorganisation [34] or endoplasmic reticulum protein trafficking [35].

Another protein with an SH2 domain that associates with the tyrosine phosphorylated PDGF receptor is the *ras* GTPase-activating protein (GAP) that attenuates signals generated by p21^{c-ras} [36]. When GAP itself is phosphorylated on tyrosines it associates with other, as yet unidentified, tyrosine phosphorylated proteins. There is so far no conclusive evidence that tyrosine phosphorylation alters the activity of PtdIns-3-kinase or GAP [11] but, conceivably, recruitment to the membrane alone is sufficient to account for their activation. The SH2 domains of PtdIns-3-kinase, GAP and PtdInsPLC-γ bind at distinct tyrosine phosphorylated sites on the PDGF receptor.

A different type of cytoplasmic protein that undergoes ligand-dependent association with the PDGF receptor is c-Raf [37]. c-Raf does not have an SH2 domain, but tyrosine phosphorylation increases its serine/threonine kinase activity. c-Raf has been reported to phosphorylate and activate another kinase, MEK, which in turn phosphorylates and activates mitogen-activated protein (MAP) kinase [38,39] (see later). Other growth factor receptor protein tyrosine kinases, including the colony stimulating factor-1 (CSF-1) receptor, EGF receptor and insulin receptor, act in a similar way to PDGF although they do not bind all 4 proteins as effectively as the PDGF-receptor and do not always cause their activation.

Oncogenes and Intracellular Signalling

Oncogene protein products produce their effects on cell proliferation and transformation by 1 of 4 possible signalling mechanisms (Fig. 3). The first is by acting as a growth factor, thus setting up an autocrine loop, for example, *fsg*-5 (FGF), *hst* (FGF) and *sis* (PDGF-B chain). The second mechanism is by acting as a protein serine/threonine or protein tyrosine kinase; *raf*, *mos*, *pks* and *rel* oncogenes fall into the first class, and *abl*, *bek* (FGF receptor), *erb* B (EGF

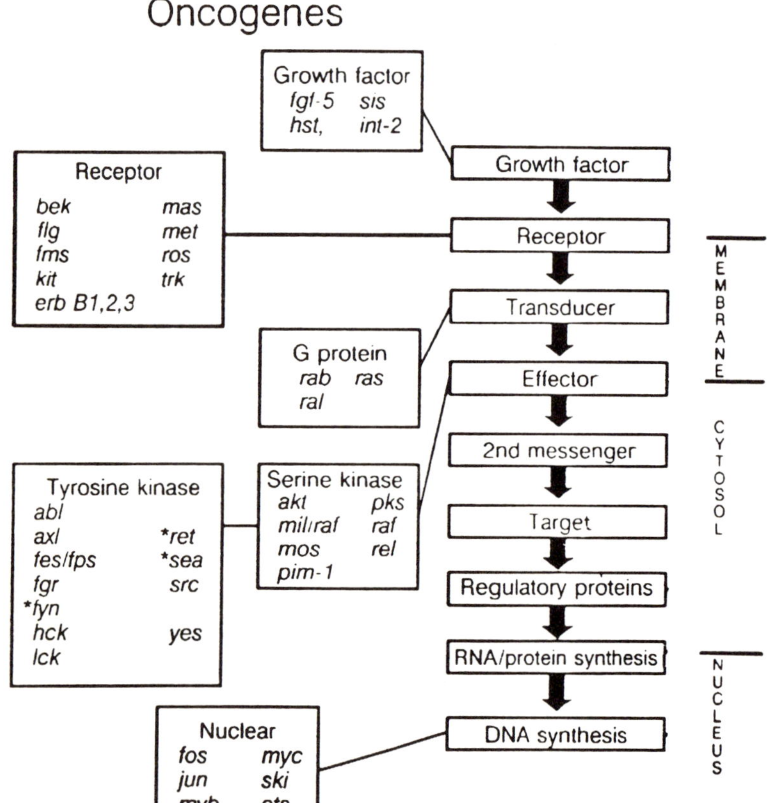

Fig. 3. Oncogenes classified by their signalling functions

receptor), *trk* (NGF receptor), *flg* (FGF receptor), *fms* (CSF-1 receptor) and *src* fall into the second class. The third mechanism involves transmission of signals by GTPases such as the protein products of *ras*, *ral*, and *rab*. The fourth mechanism is by acting as transcription regulators and includes the oncogene protein products of *erb* A, *fos*, *jun*, *myb*, *myc*, and *ski*.

Targeting the Oncogene

Oncogenes and their transcription products can be targeted directly by using antisense technology. Antisense is a term to describe any of several techniques that employs sequence-specific nucleic acid polymers to modify gene transcription or translation. The principal advantage of antisense technology over other approaches is that the mechanism of action is independent of the structural and functional characteristics of the protein to be eliminated because of the sequence specificity intrinsic to the nucleic acid interaction. Furthermore, because targeting a single gene is possible, toxicity should, in principle, be limited. The most extensively researched antisense approach is the use of antisense oligonucleotides complementary to a specific mRNA to block its translation. There remain however, considerable problems to be overcome in terms of modifying and stabilising the oligonucleotide constructs, their delivery to the cell, scale up and pharmacokinetic optimisation for human use [1,3]. Ribozymes, or RNA enzymes, mediate their own cleavage and the cleavage of RNA targets with which they hybridise at a G-U-C triplet. Since, statistically, this triplet occurs at least once in most mRNAs, a ribozyme-modified antisense RNA construct hybridising with the mRNA sequence containing the G-U-C triplet should cleave the target mRNA. While most known ribozymes bind very tightly to their targets, it is theoretically possible for each ribozyme to cleave many copies of target mRNA. However, because multiple copies of mRNA can be continually formed from a single DNA template, antisense oligonucleotides and ribozymes have to intercept a continually renewable supply of mRNA targets. Instead, by targeting DNA at the level of the gene using triple helix (triplex) technology, only a small

number of gene copies per cell have to be inhibited to block transcription [40]. Short 20 to 40 bp oligonucleotide strands can be designed that bind with high selectivity in the major groove of duplex DNA antiparallel to a purine-rich strand of the duplex. The binding affinities approach that for DNA regulatory proteins. Using the triple helix approach it is possible to selectively inhibit gene transcription in intact cells [41]. However, the selectivity of the approach for closely related genes is not known [40]. Targets under investigation using triple helix technology are *erb* B-2 and the estrogen receptor gene in breast cancer [42].

Targeting Signalling Pathways

Oncogenes or oncogene mRNA products remain, for the most part, elusive targets for drug development. Receptors and the enzymes of the growth factor signalling pathways that are activated by oncogenes are more amenable targets to pharmacologic manipulation. Some of the potential target sites are shown in Figure 4.

Inhibition of Growth Factor Receptor Binding

The earliest point at which to inhibit growth factor signalling is by preventing the binding of a growth factor to its receptor. This can be accomplished using a peptide analogue of the growth factor such as a bombesin receptor antagonist [43], or the polyanionic naphthylurea drug suramin, employed for many years to treat African trypanosomiasis and onchocerciasis, which blocks the binding of several growth factors including PDGF, TGF-ß, and EGF, to their receptors [44,45]. Other polyanionic compounds such as high molecular weight dextran sulphate, heparin and pentosan polysulphate (HOE/BAY946) have similar inhibitory effects on growth factor binding [46,47]. These compounds all exhibit antiproliferative activity against cells in culture and suramin is in clinical trial as an antitumour agent [48]. It is interesting that these polyanionic compounds also inhibit protein kinase C [49,50], PtdInsPLC and Ins(1,4,5)P$_3$ mediated Ca^{2+} release, the latter effect probably by

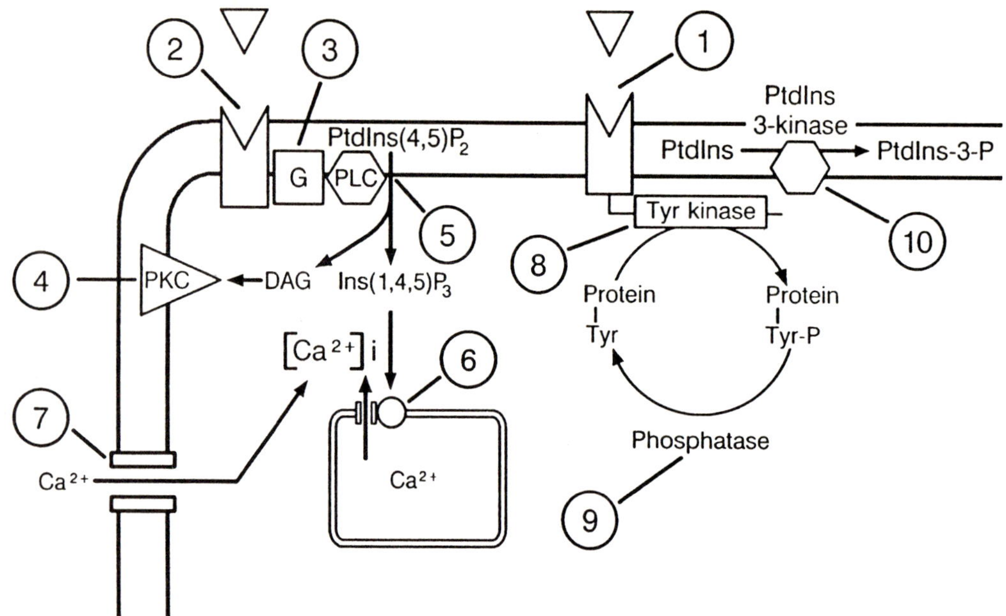

Fig 4. Target sites for modulation of growth factor signalling. 1) Inhibitors of growth factor binding; 2) mitogenic peptide antagonists; 3) inhibitors of G protein mediated enzyme activation; 4) modulators of PKC; 5) PtdInsPLC inhibitors; 6) inhibitors of the Ins(1,4,5)P₃ receptor for Ca²⁺ release; 7) inhibitors of cell membrane Ca²⁺ channels; 8) protein tyrosine kinase inhibitors; 9) modulators of phosphotyrosyl phosphates; 10) inhibitors of PtdIns-3-kinase pathway.

blocking the receptor for Ins(1,4,5)P₃ [45,51, 52].

Modulators of PKC

The PKCs are a family of 80 kDa polypeptides with a catalytic C-terminal domain and an N-terminal regulatory domain. The regulatory domain contains binding sites for Ca²⁺, phospholipid and DAG [41,53]. PKC has attracted attention as a target for cancer drug development for a number of reasons. PKC is a primary receptor for the tumour-promoting phorbol esters [24] and inhibitors of serine/threonine phosphatases mimic the effects of phorbol esters, presumably by preventing the breakdown of serine/threonine phosphorylated proteins [54]. PKC levels are altered in many tumour cells [55] and cells that overproduce PKC are susceptible to transformation by v-H-*ras* [56]. Metastatic potential has been correlated with overexpression of normal PKC [57]. Transfection with a mutant PKC gene has been reported to generate malignant and metastatic tumour cells [58], although this finding has subsequently been disputed [59]. There are at least 9 forms of PKC and 8 genes

(PKCα,ß,γ,δ,ε,ζ,η,θ) that show a different pattern of expression in wild-type and transformed cells [56,60]. Not all the forms of PKC are membrane associated or activated by Ca²⁺. As yet, no clear-cut pattern of the distribution of any of the PKC isoforms in tumour cells that might provide a selective target for drug development has emerged. Most drugs that modulate PKC activity appear to act on all the isoforms and although some selectivity of inhibition has been observed [44], this has not been extensively investigated for agents with antiproliferative activity. Some drugs that act on PKC are shown in Table 1. The nonsteroidal anti-oestrogen tamoxifen, now used increasingly in the treatment of breast cancer, and its metabolites, are inhibitors of PKC, possibly through a specific binding site at the enzyme [61]. Doxorubicin complexed with iron is a strong competitive inhibitor of PKC [62] although results in intact cells have not shown inhibition of PKC by doxorubicin [63]. The ether lipid analogues of platelet activating factor (PAF) such as 1-0-octadecyl-2-0-methyl-*rac*-glycero-3-phosphocholine (ET-18-OCH₃) can inhibit growth factor signalling at multiple sites, including inhibition of PKC [64]. An intriguing example of activation of PKC is provided by a

Table 1. Compounds acting on protein kinase C

Site of action and compound	Activity
ATP binding site	
Sangivamycin	inhibitor
Staurosporine	inhibitor
Sphingosine	inhibitor
Calphostin c	inhibitor
Regulatory site	
Doxorubicin-Fe(III)	inhibitor
Dequalinium	inhibitor
Bryostatins	partial agonist
Isoquinoline sulphonamides	inhibitor
Bisindolymaleimide	inhibitor
Aminoacridines	inhibitor
Ether lipids	inhibitor
Unknown	
Tamoxifen	inhibitor

class of macrocyclic polylactones called bryostatins [65]. The bryostatins bind to and activate PKC and show pharmacologic activity characteristic of a partial agonist. Bryostatins block the induction of cell differentiation induced by phorbol esters and can block or mimic phorbol ester's effects on cell proliferation. Translocation of PKC from the cytosol to the nuclear envelope, an effect that is not seen with phorbol esters, may help explain the bryostatin's unique activity [66]. Bryostatin 1 is currently in phase I clinical trial as an anticancer agent.

Other Serine/Threonine Kinases

Other protein serine/threonine kinases important for growth factor intracellular signalling that might provide targets for drug development are c-AMP-dependent protein kinase A (PKA) and MAP kinase. Type I PKA is thought to be important for the control of cell proliferation and type II PKA important for cell differentiation. The antiproliferative cAMP analogue 8-Cl-cAMP probably acts to restore normal gene transcription in tumour cells through an action on type II PKA [67]. MAP kinases are a group of 40 to 46 kDa protein serine/threonine kinases encoded

by the extracellular signal-regulated protein kinase (ERK) genes [18,38]. The MAP kinases appear to be critical components in the conversion of tyrosine phosphorylation signals to serine/threonine phosphorylation signals. Two protein kinases function in sequence upstream to activate MAP. One is MAP kinase-kinase or MEK, which phosphorylates MAP kinase on threonine and tyrosine regulatory sites, thus activating MAP kinase [38]. The other is c-Raf (*vide supra*) which phosphorylates and activates MEK [39]. Among the targets for phosphorylation by MAP kinase are the ribosomal S6 protein serine/threonine kinases [7] and the transcription factors c-Myc and c-Jun [53]. MAP kinases are important enzymes for transmitting growth modulating signals, particularly during the G0-G1 transition and during mitosis and meiosis [18] and could be an interesting target for pharmacologic intervention.

PtdInsPLC and Inhibitors

PtdInsPLC can be considered to be a good target for antiproliferative drugs for a number of reasons. As previously discussed, a number of growth factors and mitogens, including PDGF, EGF, and bombesin, increase PtdInsPLC activity [68]. Microinjection of PtdInsPLC-ß or PtdIns PLC-γ into quiescent NIH 3T3 cells results in dose-dependent, acute induction of DNA synthesis and spindle-shaped, highly vacuolated cells with a morphology similar to transformed cells [69]. Microinjection of antibodies against PtdInsPLC-γ, although not against PtdInsPLC-ß, into NIH 3T3 cells blocks both serum-stimulated and *ras*-stimulated DNA synthesis [70]. Mutant Chinese hamster ovary (CHO) cells lacking PIPLC-δ and with an abnormal PIPLC-γ activity do not show increased PtdIns turnover and cell proliferation in response to thrombin as do the wild-type CHO cells [71]. Breast cancer cells expressing transforming *neu*/HER2 exhibit constitutive tyrosine phosphorylation of PtdInsPLC-γ while a kinase-defective mutant of a transforming *neu*/HER2 oncogene does not mediate tyrosine phosphorylation and association with PtdInsPLC-γ [72]. Some inhibitors of PtdInsPLC are shown in Table 2. They are all cytotoxic compounds. Suramin and the ether lipid analogue ET-18-OCH$_3$ have clinical antitumour activity.

Table 2. Inhibitors of PtdInsPLC

Compound	IC$_{50}$ μM	Comments
Neomycin	10-1000	
3-nitrocoumarin	208	cytotoxic
Aminochromene	10	cytotoxic
Compound 48/80	3-8	weakly cytotoxic
U-73,122 (steroidamine)	9-40	cytotoxic, inhibits platelet aggregation
ET-18-OCH$_3$	0.4	antitumour activity
Suramin	63	antitumour activity

The ether lipid analogues are potent inhibitors of PtdInsPLC [73,74]. A number of ether lipid analogues are currently in clinical trial as antitumour agents [54,75,76]. ET-18-OCH$_3$ is a more potent inhibitor of PtdInsPLC than several other putative inhibitors of the enzyme. The inhibitory effects of ET-18-OCH$_3$ on PtdInsPLC occur at cytotoxic concentrations of the ether lipid, which first has to be incorporated into the cell membrane [77]. ET-18-OCH$_3$ inhibits cellular inositol phosphate formation caused by PDGF, and by the fluoroaluminate anion, which stimulates G protein-dependent processes. It is thus likely that ET-18-OCH$_3$ inhibits both PtdInsPLC-ß and γ [74]. ET-18-OCH$_3$ also inhibits PKC (*vide supra*) and blocks the Ins(1,4,5)P$_3$-mediated release of Ca^{2+} from intracellular stores [74]. It may be that the inhibition of intracellular signalling at several points is required for ET-18-OCH$_3$'s growth inhibitory activity.

Inhibitors of Plasma Membrane Ca^{2+} Channels

Cell membrane Ca^{2+} channels are either voltage dependent or receptor operated [78]. Inhibitors of voltage-dependent Ca^{2+} channels exhibit growth inhibitory activity against some human tumour cell lines [79,80]. L65182, a substituted carboxyimidazole originally developed as a coccidiostat which has *in vitro* and *in vivo* antitumour activity [81], inhibits intracellular signalling by blocking voltage-dependent as well as receptor-operated Ca^{2+} channels [82]. It also inhibits nucleotide biosynthesis at the level of phosphoribosyl phosphate synthetase [83] and prevents the G-protein mediated activation of PtdInsPLC [81].

PtdIns-3-Kinase Pathway

PtdIns-3-kinase is found to be associated with many growth factor receptor and oncogene protein tyrosine kinases [11]. The enzyme exists as a tightly associated heterodimer of an 85 kDa regulatory subunit and a 110 kDa catalytic subunit [84]. Evidence for a role of PtdIns-3-kinase in mitogenesis and cell transformation comes from situations where mutated tyrosine kinases fail to associate with and activate PtdIns-3-kinase. Polyoma middle T mutants that associate with and activate pp60*c-crc* tyrosine kinase but that fail to activate PtdIns-3-kinase are non-transforming [31]. The levels of cellular PtdIns-3-phosphates are elevated by transforming mutants of T but not by transformation-defective mutants [33]. Transformation-defective pp60v-*src* mutants with mutations in the *src*-homology-3 (SH3) domain, show decreased association with PtdIns-3-kinase [40]. Cells transfected with mutant PDGF receptors that retain protein tyrosine kinase activity but that do not associate with or activate PtdIns-3-kinase, fail to show a mitogenic response to PDGF, unlike cells transfected with the wild-type PDGF receptor [85]. A transforming Neu/HER2 oncoprotein is found constitutively coupled to PtdIns-3-kinase while non-transforming kinase-defective or carboxyl-terminal deleted versions show no constitutive association with PtdIns-3-kinase [86]. A mutant CSF-1 receptor with a kinase-insert deletion shows a significantly reduced association with PtdIns-3-kinase and, while it is capable of conferring CSF-1-dependent transformation to some cells, it has lost the ability in other cells [28,87]. The only reported inhibitors of PtdIns-3-kinase are quercetin and some of its analogues [88], together with ET-18-OCH$_3$ and some other antitumour ether lipids [89]. Both classes of compounds are relatively non-specific inhibitors of PtdIns-3-kinase and will also block other signalling enzymes [64,74,90,91]. We have been studying a series of D-3-deoxy-3-substituted *myo*-inositol analogues that can be incorporated into PtdIns, and appear to act as *myo*-inositol antimetabolites in the PtdIns-3-phosphate signalling pathway [92].

The D-3-deoxy-3-substituted *myo*-inositol analogues exhibit growth inhibitory activity that is selective for v-*sis* transformed NIH 3T3 cells compared to wild-type NIH 3T3 cells. The most potent analogues are D-3-deoxy-3-chloro-*myo*-inositol, IC_{50} for v-*sis* NIH 3T3 cells 0.39 mM, and D-3-deoxy-3-azido-*myo*-inositol, IC_{50} 0.04 mM [93,94]. The growth inhibitory activity of the analogues is, as is expected for an antimetabolite, antagonised by *myo*-inositol, but this antagonism occurs even at physiological concentrations (40 µM) of *myo*-inositol. Thus, the analogues themselves are unlikely to be useful *in vivo* antitumour agents and more potent derivatives are needed. In order to circumvent the antagonism of the *myo*-inositol analogues by *myo*-inositol, we are investigating synthetic PtdIns containing D-3-deoxy-3-substituted *myo*-inositol, that should bypass the uptake and synthesis into PtdIns, where we believe the competition by *myo*-inositol occurs [92]. The first of the PtdIns's we have studied, D-3-deoxy-3-fluoro-PtdIns, exhibited growth inhibitory activity against wild type NIH 3T3 and v-*sis* transformed NIH 3T3 cells with IC_{50}s of 100 µM. *myo*-Inositol in the medium has no effect on growth inhibition by the compound. The mechanism of inhibition of cell growth by D-3-deoxy-3-fluoro-PtdIns remains to be established.

Inhibitors of Protein Tyrosine Kinases

A number of growth factor receptors when activated by the appropriate ligand are protein tyrosine kinases [4,95]. They include the receptors for PDGF, EGF, CSF-1 and insulin. There are also a large number of non-receptor and receptor-like oncogenic protein tyrosine kinases [11]. Tyrosine phosphorylated proteins are known to be important mediators of cell proliferation [96]. Selective inhibition of these protein tyrosine kinases could, theoretically, lead to inhibition of cell proliferation and even the reversal of transformation, and considerable effort is currently being devoted to developing this class of inhibitors. Some examples of inhibitors and their relative selectivity for different protein tyrosine kinases are given in Table 3. The ATP binding region is conserved in many protein tyrosine kinases and inhibitors that act at this site, such as the bioflavonoids genistein and quercetin [90], may have too broad a

Table 3. Inhibitors of protein tyrosine kinase

Site of action and compound	Protein tyrosine kinase inhibited[a]
ATP binding site	
Bioflavonoid	EGF-R, I-R, *src, fes, fps*
Lavendustin A	EGF-R
Amiloride	EGF-R, I-R, PDGF-R
Staurosporine	PDGF-R, I-R, > EGF-R
Doxorubicin	*abl*
Peptide site	
Erbstatins	EGF-R > PAF-R, *src* > I-R
Tyrphostins	EGF-R, PDGF-R, *src, abl* > PAF-R > I-R[b]
Cinnamamides	EGF-R, *fgr* > *fos, src*
Piceatannol	p40 > lck
Unknown mechanism	
Herbimycin A	*src*, abl
Thiazolidinediones	EGF-R, *src* > abl
Sulphonylbenzoyl nitrostyroles	EGF-R
Chlorpromazine	*src*
(+)-Aeroplysinin-1	EGF-R

[a] R = receptor; I = insulin; PAF = platelet activating factor
[b] Specificity depends on the analogue

specificity to be useful inhibitors of protein tyrosine kinases. Genistein is also an inhibitor of DNA topoisomerase II [91]. Amiloride, an inhibitor of the Na^+/H^+ antiporter, is also an inhibitor of receptor protein tyrosine kinases, competitive with ATP, at concentrations that are cytotoxic to cells [38]. Doxorubicin at relatively high (50 to 100 µM) concentrations can inhibit protein tyrosine kinases [39]. Erbstatin, isolated originally from an actinomycete broth, is a tyrosine analogue that blocks the peptide site of the EGF-receptor and *src* protein tyrosine kinases [97]. Erbstatin also inhibits DNA topoisomerases I and II [98]. *In vitro* erbastatin inhibits EGF-dependent cell proliferation and *in vivo* has antitumour activity against murine L1210 leukaemia and against human mammary carcinoma growing in athymic nude mice, [99,100]. The usefulness of erbastatin may be limited by its degradation by ferric or ferrous iron present in serum [100]. The tyrphostins are a series of compounds related to erbstatin. They inhibit EGF-receptor and PDGF-receptor tyrosine kinase activity in intact cells at concentrations that also inhibit EGF- and PDGF-dependent DNA synthesis and cell proliferation [101]. Considerably higher concentrations of tyrphostins are required to inhibit serum-dependent cell proliferation [102]. Hydroxycinnamide derivatives inhibit protein tyrosine kinase probably because of their similarity to tyrosine [103]. Herbimycin A, a benzoquinoid ansamycin antibiotic, inhibits *v-src* protein tyrosine kinase [104]. It blocks the growth of *v-src* transformed cells and reverses their transformed phenotype, which is how herbimycin A's activity was originally discovered. Imipramine, chlorpromazine, dibucaine and tetracaine are weak inhibitors of *src* protein tyrosine kinase, probably by interaction with a phospholipid binding site [18]. The development of tyrosine kinase inhibitors is reviewed in more detail in the chapter by Workman (see also [105]).

Strategies for Developing Signalling Drugs

After having established a suitable and sensitive *in vitro* biochemical assay for the signalling target under investigation, compounds have to be screened to find potent inhibitors. There are at least 4 potential sources of new compounds for screening, 1) random screening of plant and animal extracts and microbiological fermentation broths, 2) random screening of off-the-shelf chemical compounds, 3) chemical modification of previously identified active compounds, and 4) model-directed synthesis of compounds based on a detailed knowledge of the unique structural features and activity of the protein target in question. The latter route to new compounds, although intellectually most satisfying, is probably some years away for most targets we can identify. In the near future, the random screening of natural extracts and synthetic chemicals is likely to yield the greatest return in terms of novel lead compounds. These compounds can then, if necessary, be chemically modified to improve their activity and provide structure activity information about the target. For example, with most biochemical screens access of the compound to the target is not a problem. Active agents identified by these screens may not penetrate the intact cell and may have to be chemically modified to improve bioavailability. The choice of appropriate *in vitro* and *in vivo* biological models to demonstrate antitumour activity also presents problems. It can be argued that since the available tumour models have failed to identify sufficiently active and selective anticancer drugs from the hundreds of thousands of compounds that have already been tested, they may not be the most appropriate models for demonstrating the antitumour activity of new classes of compounds. At the very least, it seems that growth in the tumour model being used should depend upon the signalling target studied. For example, when using an oncogene or oncoprotein as the drug target, the oncogene should be known to be expressed in the tumour model and should contribute to its proliferation.

To adequately test the hypothesis that growth factor and oncogene signalling pathways offer target sites for anticancer drug development, the drugs developed by the approach have to be tested in patients. This process takes several years and we are unable to say at this time whether the approach will work. There are, however, a small number of compounds in the early stages of clinical development as anticancer agents that may act by inhibiting growth factor signalling pathways. In all cases the activity of the compounds on intracellular signalling pathways was discovered after their identification as antiproliferative agents. There are also compounds in preclinical development that have been specifically developed as inhibitors of growth factor signalling, although their selectivity for tumour cells compared to normal tissue remains to be fully investigated in animal tumour models. The drugs need to be tested in appropriate animal models and clinical subjects. This means that the tumour should be shown to express the oncogene or signalling pathway that is to be inhibited. It may be more appropriate, for the type of drugs considered here, to classify tumours by their complement of oncogenes and tumour suppressor genes, rather than by their histopathological type. As discussed previously, it is possible that a single drug by itself may not have the power to completely inhibit tumour growth and a combination of drugs may be needed. It may also take a combination of drugs to prevent the emergence of resistance.

Clearly there are several challenges, and there will undoubtedly be others, that have to be faced in developing this new class of anti-cancer drugs.

Acknowledgements

Work described conducted in the author's laboratory was supported by NIH Grants CA 42286 and CA 52995. The excellent secretarial assistance of Ms Madelon Cook and Ms Janel Janssen is gratefully acknowledged.

REFERENCES

1   Einhorn J: Nitrogen mustard: the origin of chemotherapy in cancer. Int J Rad Oncol Phys 1985 (2):1375-1378
2   Anonymous: Facts and Comparisons. JB Lippincott, St Louis 1992
3   DeVita VT: Principles of chemotherapy in cancer. In: DeVita VT, Hellman S and Rosenberg SA (eds) Principles and Practice of Oncology. JB Lippincott, Philadelphia 1989 pp 276-300
4   Heidelberger C, Chaudhari NK, Danneberg, Mooren D, Griesbach L, Duchinsky R, Schnitze RJ, Pleven E and Scheiner J: Fluorinated pyrimidines. A new class of tumour-inhibitory compounds. Nature 1957 (179):663-666
5   Boyd MR: Status of implementation of the NCI human tumor cell line in vitro primary drug screen. Proc Am Assoc Cancer Res 1989 (30):652
6   Travali S, Koniecki J, Petralia S and Baserga R: Oncogenes in growth and development. FASEB J 1990 (4):3209-3214
7   Hollingsworth RE and Lee W-H: Tumor suppressor genes: New prospects for cancer research. JNCI 1991 (83):91-96
8   Marx J: Possible new colon cancer gene found. Science 1991 (251):1317-1318
9   Lucibelio FC and Muller R: Transcription factor encoding oncogenes. Rev Physiol Biochem Pharmacol 1992 (119):225-257
10   Deuel TF: Polypeptide growth factors: Roles in normal and abnormal cell growth. Annu Rev Cell Biol 1987 (3):443-492
11   Cantley LC, Auger KR, Carpenter C, Duckworth B, Graziani A, Kapeller R and Soltoff S: Oncogenes and signal transduction. Cell 1991 (64):281-302
12   Soriano P, Montgomery C, Geske R and Bradley A: Targeted disruption of the c-*src* proto-oncogene leads to osteoporosis in mice. Cell 1991 (64):693-702
13   Macara IG: Oncogenes and cellular signal transduction. Physiol Rev 1989 (69):797-820
14   Smith MR, DeGudicibus SJ and Stacey DW: Requirement for c-*ras* proteins during viral oncogene transformation. Nature 1986 (320):540-543
15   Helene C: Rational design of sequence-specific oncogene inhibitors based on antisense and antigene oligonucleotides. Eur J Cancer 1991 (27):1466-1477
16   Kashani-Sabet M, Funato T, Tone T et al: Reversal of the malignant phenotype by an anti-*ras* ribozyme. Antisense Research and Development 1992 (2):3-15
17   Albino AP, LeStrange R, Oliff AI, Furth ME and Old LJ: Transforming ras genes from human melanoma: a manifestation of tumour heterogeneity? Nature 1984 (308):69-72
18   Thomas G: MAP kinase by any other name smells just as sweet. Cell 1992 (68):3-6
19   Tannock IF: Experimental chemotherapy. In: Tannock IF and Hill RP (eds) The Basic Science of Oncology. Pergamon Press, New York 1992 pp 308-325
20   Tannock IF: Tumor growth and cell kinetics. In: Tannock IF and Hill RP (eds) The Basic Science of Oncology. Pergamon Press, New York 1987 pp 140-159
21   Mihich E and Ehrke MJ: Immunomodulation by anticancer drugs. In: DeVita VT, Hellman S and Rosenberg SA (eds) Biologic Therapy of Cancer. JB Lippincott, Philadelphia 1991 pp 776-786
22   Smrcka AV, Hepler JR, Brown KO and Sternweis PC: Regulation of polyphosphoinositide-specific phospholipase C activity by purified G_q. Science 1990 (251):804
23   Berridge MJ and Irvine RF: Inositol phosphates and cell signalling. Nature 1989 (341):197-205
24   Kikkawa U and Nishizuka Y: The role of protein kinase C in transmembrane signalling. Annu Rev Cell Biol 1986 (2):149-178
25   Irvine RF, Moore RM, Pollock WK, Smith PM and Wreggett KA: Inositol phosphates: proliferation, metabolism and function. Philos Trans R Soc Lond B 1988 (320):281-298
26   Irvine RF and Moore RM: Microinjection of inositol 1,3,4,5-tetrakisphosphate activates sea urchin eggs by a mechanism dependent on external Ca^{2+}. Biochem J 1986 (240):917-920
27   Bishayee S, Majumdar S, Khire J and Das M: Ligand-induced dimerization of the platelet-derived growth factor receptor. J Biol Chem 1989 (264): 11699-11705
28   Nishimura J, Huang JS and Deuel TF: Platelet-derived growth factor stimulates tyrosine specific protein kinase activity in Swiss mouse 3T3 cell membranes. Proc Natl Acad Sci USA 1982 (79):4303-4307
29   Moran MF, Koch CA, Anderson D, Ellis C, England L, Martin GC and Pawson T: Src homology region 2 domains direct protein-protein interactions in signal transduction. Proc Natl Acad Sci USA 1990 (87):8622-8626 (abstract)
30   Wahl MI, Oleshaw NE, Nishibe B, Rhee SG, Pledger WJ and Carpenter G: Platelet-derived growth factor induces rapid and sustained tyrosine phosphorylation of phospholipase C-gamma in quiescent BALB/c 3T3 cells. Mol Cell Biol 1989 (9):2934-2943
31   Kaplan DR, Whitman M, Schaffhausen B, Pallas DC, White M, Cantley L and Roberts TM: Common elements in growth factor stimulation and

oncogenic transformation: 85 kd phosphoprotein and phosphatidylinositol kinase activity. Cell 1987 (50):1021-1029

32 Downes CP and Carter AN: Phosphoinositide 3-kinase: a new effector in signal transduction? Cell Signalling 1991 (3):501

33 Serunian LA, Auger KR, Roberts T and Cantley LC: Production of novel polyphosphoinositides in vivo is linked to cell transformation by polyomavirus middle T antigen. J Virol 1989 (64):4718-4725

34 Eberle M, Traynor-Kaplan AE, Sklar LA and Norgauer J: Is there a relationship between phosphatidylinositol trisphosphate and F-actin polymerization in human neutrophils? J Biol Chem 1990 (265):16725-16728

35 Hiles ID, Otsu M, Volinia S et al: Phosphotidylinositol 3-kinase: structure and expression of the 110 kd catalytic subunit. Cell 1992 (70):419

36 McCormick F: The world according to GAP. Oncogene 1990 (5):1281-1287

37 Morrison DK, Kaplan DR, Rapp U and Roberts TM: Signal transduction from membrane to cytoplasm: growth factors and membrane-bound oncogene products increase Raf-1 phosphorylation and associated protein kinase activity. Proc Natl Acad Sci USA 1988 (85):8855-8859

38 Crews CM, Alessandrini A and Erikson RL: The primary structure of MEK, a protein kinase that phosphorylates the ERK gene product. Science 1992 (258):478-480

39 Kyriakis JM, App H, Zang X-f et al: Raf-1 activates MAP kinase-kinase. Nature 1992 (358):417-419

40 Chubb JM and Hogen ME: Human therapeutics based on triple helix technology. Trends Biotech 1992 (10):132-136

41 Postel E, Flint SJ, Kessler DJ and Hogan ME: Evidence that a triplex-forming oligodeoxyribonucleotide binds to the c-myc mRNA levels. Proc Natl Acad Sci USA 1991 (88):8227-8331

42 Gazit A, Yaish P, Gilon C and Levitzki A: Tyrphostins I: Synthesis and biological activity of protein tyrosine kinase inhibitors. J Med Chem 1989 (32):2344

43 Trepel JB, Moyer JD, Cuttitta F et al: A novel bombesin receptor antagonist inhibits autocrine signals in a small cell lung carcinoma cell line. Biochem Biophys Res Commun 1988 (156):1383-1389

44 Coffey RJ, Leof EB, Shipley GD and Moses HL: Suramin inhibition of growth factor receptor binding and mitogenicity in AKR-2B cells. J Cell Physiol 1987 (132):143-148

45 Seewald JM, Olsen RA and Powis G: Suramin blocks intracellular Ca^{2+} release and growth factor-induced increases in cytoplasmic free Ca^{2+} concentration. Cancer Lett 1989 (49):107-113

46 Powis G, Seewald MJ, Sehgal I, Iaizzo PA and Olsen RA: Platelet-derived growth factor stimulates non-mitochondrial Ca^{2+} uptake and inhibits mitogen-induced Ca^{2+} signalling in Swiss 3T3 fibroblasts. J Biol Chem 1990 (82):167-168

47 Newman ME: AIDS drug gets trial as cancer therapy. JNCI 1990 (82):167-168

48 LaRocca RV, Stein CA and Myers CE: Suramin: prototype of a new generation of antitumour compounds. Cancer Cells 1990 (2):106-115

49 Hensey CE, Boscoboinik D and Azzi A: Suramin, an anticancer drug, inhibits protein kinase C and induces differentiation in neuroblastoma cell clone NB2A. FEBS Lett 1989 (258):156-158

50 Herbert JM and Maffrand JP: Effect of pentosan polysulphate, standard heparin and related compounds on protein kinase C activity. Biochim Biophys Acta 1991 (1091):432-441

51 Seewald MJ, Olsen R, Melder D and Powis G: High molecular weight dextran sulfate inhibits intracellular Ca^{2+} release and decreases growth factor induced increases in intracellular free Ca^{2+} in Swiss 3T3 fibroblasts. Cancer Commun 1989 (1):151-156

52 Tones MA, Bootman MD, Higgins BF, Lane DA, Pay GF and Lindahl U: The effect of heparin on the inositol 1,4,5-trisphosphate receptor in rat liver microsomes. FEBS Lett 1989 (252):105-108

53 Alvarez E, Northwood IC, Gonzalez FA, Latour DA, Seth A, Abate C, Curran T and Davis RJ: Pro-Leu-Ser/Thr-Pro is a consensus primary sequence for substrate protein phosphorylation. Characterization of the phosphorylation of c-myc and c-jun proteins by an epidermal growth factor receptor threonine 669 protein kinase. J Biol Chem 1991 (266):15377-15285

54 Suganuma M, Fijiki H, Surguri H et al: Okadaic acid: an additional non-phorbol-12-tetradecanoate-13-acetatetype tumor promoter. Proc Natl Acad Sci USA 1988 (85):1768-1771

55 Barr LF, Mabry M, Nelkin BD, Tyrler G, May WS and Baylin SB: c-myc gene induced alterations in protein kinase C expression: A possible mechanism facilitating myc-ras gene complementation. Cancer Res 1991 (51):5514-5519

56 Borner C, Guadagno SN, Hsieh LL, Hsiao WL and Weinstein IB: Transformation by a ras oncogene causes increased expression of protein kinase C-alpha and decreased expression of protein kinase C-epsilon. Cell Growth Differ 1990 (1):653-660

57 Housey GM, Johnson MD, Hsias WLW et al: Overproduction of protein kinase C causes disordered growth control in rat fibroblasts. Cell 1988 (52):343-354

58 Megedish T and Mazurek N: A mutant protein kinase C that can transform fibroblasts. Nature 1989 (324):807-811

59 Borner C, Filipuzzi I, Weinstein IB and Imber L: Failure of wild-type of a mutant form of protein kinase C-alpha to transform fibroblasts. Nature 1991 (353):78-83

60 Nixon JS, Bishop J, Bradshaw D et al: The design and biological properties of potent and selective inhibitors of protein kinase C. Biochem Soc Trans 1992 (20):419-425

61 O'Brian CA, Housey GM and Weinstein IB: Specific and direct binding of protein kinase C to an immobilized tamoxifen analogue. Cancer Res 1988 (48):3626

62 Hannun YA, Fogleson RJ and Bell RM: The adriamycin-iron (III) complex is a potent inhibitor of

protein kinase C. J Biol Chem 1989 (264):9960-9966

63 Otsuka M, Shigeoka H and Yang HC: In vivo effects of doxorubicin on kinase C in cultured cells. Cancer Chemother Pharmacol 1992 (30):407-411

64 Helfman DM, Barnes KC, Kinkade JM, Vogler WR, Shoji MM and Kuo JF: Phospholipid-sensitive Ca^{2+} dependent protein phosphorylation system in various types of leukemic cells from human patients and in human leukemic cell lines HL60 and K562, and its inhibition by alkyl-lysophospholipid. Cancer Res 1983 (43):2955-2961

65 Jones RJ, Sharkis SJ, Miller CB, Rowinsky EK, Burke PJ and May WS: Bryostatin 1, a unique biologic response modifier: Anti-leukemic activity in vitro. Blood 1990 (75):1319-1323

66 Gescher A and Dale IL: Protein kinase C - a novel target for rational anticancer drug design? Anti-Cancer Drug Design 1989 (4):93-105

67 Cho-Chung YS: Site-selective 8-chloro-cyclic adenosine 3',5'-monophosphate as a biologic modulator of cancer: Restoration of normal control mechanisms. JNCI 1989 (81):982-987

68 Nanberg E and Rozengurt E: Temporal relationship between inositol polyphosphate formation and increases in cytosolic Ca^{2+} in quiescent 3T3 cells stimulated by platelet-derived growth factor, bombesin and vasopressin. EMBO J 1988 (7):2741-2747

69 Smith MR, Ryu SH, Suh PG, Rhee SG and Kung HF: S-phase induction and transformation of quiescent NIH 3T3 cells by microinjection of phospholipase C. Proc Natl Acad Sci USA 1989 (86):3659-3663 (abstract)

70 Smith MR, Liu Y-L, Kim H, Rhee SG and Kung HF: Inhibition of serum- and *ras*-stimulated DNA synthesis by antibodies to phospholipase C. Science 1990 (247):1074-1077

71 Rath HM, Doyle GAR and Silbert DF: Hamster fibroblasts defective in thrombin-induced mitogenesis. J Biol Chem 1989 (264):13387-13390

72 Peles E, Levy RB, Or E, Ullrich A and Yarden Y: Oncogenic forms of the *neu*/HER2 tyrosine kinase are permanently coupled to phospholipase C gamma. EMBO J 1991 (10):2077

73 Überall F, Oberhuber H, Maly K, Zaknun J, Demuth L and Grunicke HH: Hexadecylphosphocholine inhibits inositol phosphate formation and protein kinase C activity. Cancer Res 1991 (51):807-812

74 Carpenter CL and Cantley LC: Phosphoinositide kinases. Biochemistry 1990 (29):11147-11155

75 Berdel WE, Schlehe H, Fink U et al: Early tumor and leukemia response to alkyl-lysophospholipids in a phase I study. Cancer 1982 (50):2011

76 Herrmann DBJ, Neumann HA, Heim ME et al: Short- and long-term tolerability study of the thioether phospholipid derivative ilmofosine in cancer patients. Contrib Oncol 1989 (37):236-247

77 Powis G, Seewald MJ, Melder D, Hoke M and Olsen R: Inhibition of growth factor receptor binding and cell growth inhibition by sulfonated azo dyes: comparison with the antitumor agent suramin. Cancer Res 1992 (31):223-228

78 Putney JW Jr: Receptor-regulated calcium entry. Pharmacol Ther 1990 (48):427-434

79 Schmidt WF, Huber KR, Ettinger RS and Neuberg RW: Antiproliferative effect of verapamil alone on brain tumor cells in vitro. Cancer Res 1988 (48):3617-3621

80 Worley JF and Strobl JS: Voltage-dependent calcium channels in MCF-7 human breast cancer cells and inhibition of cell growth by calcium channel antagonists. Cancer Chemother Pharmacol 1989 (24):S84 (abstract)

81 Kohn EC and Liotta A: L651582: A novel antiproliferative and antimetastasis agent. JNCI 1990 (82):54-60

82 Hupe DJ, DiSalvo J and Schaeffer MR: A novel antiproliferative and antimetastasis agent which interferes with calcium signal transduction. Cancer Chemother Pharmacol 1989 (24):S85 (abstract)

83 Hupe DJ, Behrens ND and Boltz R: Anti-proliferative activity of L-651,582 correlates with calcium-mediated regulation of nucleotide metabolism at phosphoribosyl pyrophosphate synthetase. J Cell Physiol 1990 (144):457-466

84 Shibaski F, Homma Y and Takenawa T: Monomer and heterodimer forms of phosphatidylinositol-3-kinase. J Biol Chem 1991 (266):8108

85 Coughlin SR, Escobedo JA and Williams LT: Role of phosphatidylinositol kinase in PDGF receptor signal transduction. Science 1989 (243):1191-1194

86 Peles E, Lamprecht R, Ben-Levy R, Tzahar E and Yarden Y: Regulated coupling of the Neu receptor to phosphatidylinositol 3'-kinase and its release by oncogenic activation. J Biol Chem 1992 (267):12266-12274

87 Shurtleff SA, Downing JR, Rock CO, Hawkins SA, Roussel MF and Sherr CJ: Structural features of the colony-stimulating factor 1 receptor that affect its association with phosphatidylinositol 3-kinase. EMBO J 1990 (9):2415-2421

88 Matter WF, Brown RF and Vlahos CJ: The inhibition of phosphatidylinositol 3-kinase by quercetin and analogs. Biochem Biophys Res Commun 1992 (186):624-631

89 Augustine J, Berggren M, Powis G and Modest E: Inhibition of phosphatidylinositol-3'-kinase by ether lipid analogue of phosphatidylinositol and phosphatidylcholine. Proc Am Assoc Cancer Res 1992 (33):415

90 Akiyama T, Ishida J, Nakagawa S, Ogawara H, Watanabe S, Itoh N, Shibuya M and Fukami Y: Genistein, a specific inhibitor of tyrosine-specific protein kinases. J Biol Chem 1987 (262):5592-5595

91 Markovits J, Linassier C, Fosse P, Couprie J, Pierre J, Jacquemin-Sablon A, Saucier JM, Le-Pecq JB and Larsen AK: Inhibitory effects of the tyrosine kinase inhibitor genistein on mammalian DNA topoisomerase II. Cancer Res 1989 (49):5111-5117

92 Brunn G, Fauq AH, Chow S, Kozikowski AP, Gallegos A and Powis G: Cellular pharmacology of D-3-deoxy-*myo*-inositol, an inhibitor of phosphatidylinositol signalling having antiproliferative activity. Proc Natl Acad Sci USA 1992 (in press)

93 Fauq AH, Kozikowski AP, Powis G and Melder DC: D-3-modified myo-inositol analogues: synthesis and growth inhibitory properties. J Med Chem 1991 (in press)

94   Powis G, Aksoy IA, Melder DC, Aksoy S, Eichinger H, Fauq AH and Kozikowski AP: D-3-deoxy-substituted myo-inositol analogues as inhibitors of cell growth. Cancer Chemother Pharmacol 1991 (29):95-104

95   Ullrich A and Schlesinger J: Signal transduction by receptors with tyrosine kinase activity. Cell 1990 (61):203-212

96   Glenney JR Jr: Tyrosine-phosphorylated proteins: mediators of signal transduction from the tyrosine kinases. Biochim Biophys Acta 1992 (1134):113-127

97   Umezawa H, Imoto M, Sawa T, Isshiki K, Matsuda N, Uchida T, Iinuma H, Hamada M and Takeuchi T: Studies on a new epidermal growth factor-receptor kinase inhibitor, erbstatin, produced by MH435-hF3. J Antibiot 1986 (39):170-173

98   Markovits J, Saucier JM, Larsen AR, Mendoza R, Jacquemin-Sablon A, Le Pecq JB and Umezawa K: Effect of the tyrosine kinase inhibitor, erbstatin, on DNA topoisomerases. Proc Am Assoc Cancer Res 1990 (31):439 (abstract)

99   Imoto M, Umezawa K, Komuro K, Sawa T, Takeuchi T and Umezawa H: Antitumor activity of erbstatin, a tyrosine protein kinase inhibitor. Jpn J Cancer Res 1987 (78):329-332

100   Toi M, Mukaida H, Wada T, Hirabayashi N, Toge T, Hori T and Umezawa K: Antineoplastic effect of erbstatin on human mammary and esophageal tumors in athymic nude mice. Eur J Cancer 1990 (26):722-724

101   Levitzki A and Gilon C: Tyrphostins as molecular tools and potential antiproliferative drugs. Trends Pharmacol Sci 1991 (12):171-176

102   Lyall RM, Zilbertstein A, Gazit A, Gilon C, Levitzki A and Schlessinger J: Tyrphostins inhibit epidermal growth factor (EGF)-receptor tyrosine kinase activity in living cells and EGF-stimulated cell proliferation. J Biol Chem 1989 (264):14503-14509

103   Shiraishi T, Owada MK, Tatsuka M, Yamashita T, Watanabe K and Kakunaga T: Specific inhibitors of tyrosine-specific protein kinases: Properties of 4-hydroxycinnamamide derivatives in vitro. Cancer Res 1989 (49):2374-2378

104   Uehara Y, Fukazawa H, Murakami Y and Mizuno S: Irreversible inhibition of v-*src* tyrosine kinase activity by herbimycin A and its abrogation by sulphydryl compounds. Biochem Biophys Res Commun 1989 (163):803-809

105   Workman P, Brunton V and Robins R: Tyrosine kinase inhibitors. Sem Cancer Biol 1992 (3):369-381

Discovery and Design of Inhibitors of Oncogenic Tyrosine Kinases

Paul Workman [1], Valerie G. Brunton [1] and David J. Robins [2]

1 Cancer Research Campaign Department of Medical Oncology, University of Glasgow, CRC Beatson Laboratories, Garscube Estate, Switchback Road, Bearsden, Glasgow G61 1BD
2 Department of Chemistry, University of Glasgow, Glasgow G12 8QQ, United Kingdom

The recognition that we may be approaching a plateau of effectiveness with traditional anticancer agents has led to the view that to gain more than incremental value against the major solid tumours will require a radically different strategy. Rather than the "black box" approach of random screening for cytotoxicity or cytostasis, or even the rational design of improved agents acting on conventional drug targets [1,2], many believe that this quantum leap will come from an exploitation of the identification of the genes and their encoded protein products which control proliferation, differentiation and cell death, combined with an understanding of their aberrant behaviour in malignant cells. Cancer is now described in extraordinary detail at the molecular level as a genetic disease. As a result of the remarkable advances in molecular oncology made over the last few years, the new central dogma of cancer drug discovery can be defined as: new biology → new targets → new therapies [3].

Genetic instability is an invariant hallmark of cancer cells, and human oncogenesis is known to be associated with, and indeed driven by, an accumulation of genetic abnormalities. This process is particularly well defined in human colorectal cancer [4], but a similar molecular description is now emerging for a range of other human tumour types. If cancer cell growth can be likened to an out of control motor car, then the mutation or increased expression of oncogenes is equivalent to a recklessly sustained pressure on the accelerator pedal, while the mutation and loss of tumour suppressor genes can be likened to a faulty brake pedal. The challenge for innovative drug discovery is to identify specific inhibitors of oncogene pathways or to find means of replacing lost suppressor functions. The latter is clearly more difficult than the former. It is now certain that all oncogenes and tumour suppressor genes encode proteins which are involved in signal transduction: either as components in growth factor signalling pathways or as key players in the regulation of DNA fidelity, cell cycle control, and programmed cell death or apoptosis. Thus at the protein level cancer can be viewed as a disease of faulty signal transduction and the signalling proteins themselves represent excellent targets for the discovery of new anticancer agents [5,6]. In addition, the signals involved in angiogenesis, invasion and metastasis are also very attractive. The promise and potential problems of the overall approach are reviewed in the previous chapter by Powis.

Of the many signal transduction mechanisms which are emerging as potential targets for drug hunting in cancer, the tyrosine kinase activities associated with growth factor receptors and oncogene products are receiving particular attention from both pharmaceutical companies and academic groups. For previous reviews of the area the reader is referred to references 7-13.

Protein kinases are vital for all aspects of cell function. There are at least 200 of these enzymes and up to a thousand have been predicted [14]. They catalyse the transfer of the γ-phosphate of ATP (or in some cases GTP) in general to either serine/threonine or tyrosine residues located within a particular peptide sequence in the protein substrate (Fig. 1). While serine/threonine kinases, particularly protein kinase C, are also targets for drug development [15,16], we will focus here on tyrosine kinases, of which over 40 vertebrate forms are now known [11].

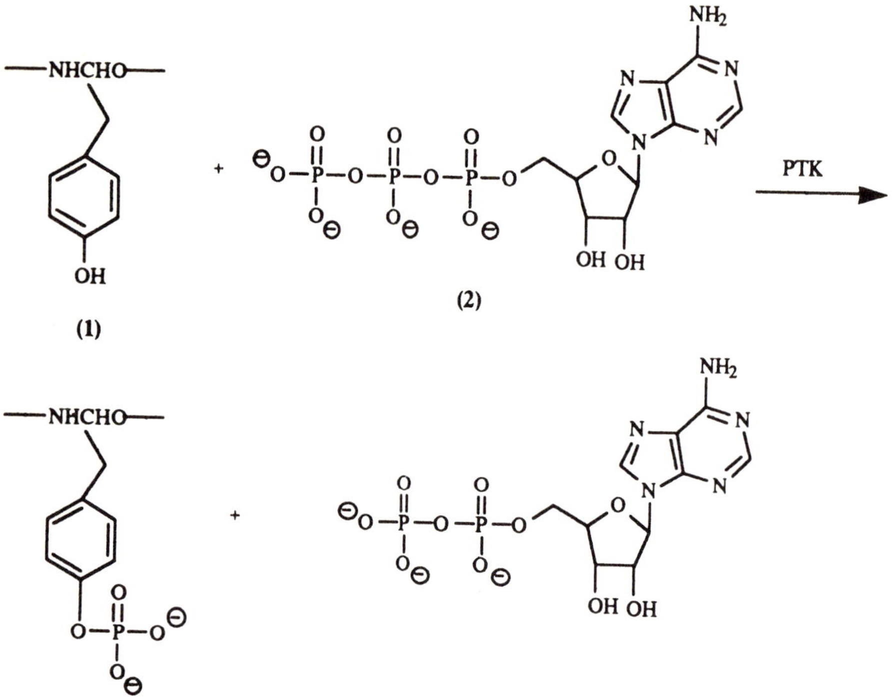

Fig. 1. The chemical reaction catalysed by tyrosine kinases. The γ phosphate group of ATP is transferred to tyrosine hydroxyl located within the protein substrate. This usually acts as a molecular signal by modifying the activity of the protein substrate or its ability to bind protein partners.

A relatively small proportion of phosphorylated residues on proteins involve tyrosine, and the amount is kept in close check by the opposing effects of tyrosine kinases and tyrosine phosphatases. When cellular tyrosine phosphorylation is increased by the appropriate stimulus (for example the docking of cognate ligand to a cell membrane receptor or the mutation or increased expression of a particular oncogene), this initiates a cascade of downstream biochemical events, many of which involve sequential protein phosphorylation and protein-protein interactions [see later and ref. 17]. The biological outcome can take the form of a variety of cellular responses, the nature of which can vary with both the stimulus and the cell type.

Tyrosine Kinases and Cancer

The tyrosine kinases can be divided into 2 categories: those associated with the cytosolic domains of cell membrane receptors, and those that are non-receptor tyrosine kinases. Examples of the former are the so-called class 1 receptor tyrosine kinases, including the epidermal growth factor (EGF) and c-erbB2 (HER2 or neu) receptors [17] which are often overexpressed in human tumours such as breast and ovarian cancers. Moreover, this increased expression, sometimes associated with gene amplification, can be an important prognostic factor in these settings [18,19]. Although this does not necessarily prove a causal relationship, it is nevertheless very strong evidence that tyrosine kinase activity does contribute to the growth of these cancers. Other receptor tyrosine kinases which are overexpressed in human malignancy include those for platelet-derived growth factor (PDGF) and the fibroblast growth factors (FGFs) [17]. In addition to their mitogenic action, the FGFs, together with vascular endothelial growth factor (VEGF), are also implicated in tumour angiogenesis [20].

Examples of non-receptor tyrosine kinases (which nevertheless do associate with the cell membrane) include c-src which shows increased activity in colon, breast and other tumours [21,22]. In patients with chronic myelogenous leukaemia, the translocation involving chromosomes 9 and 22 results in the fusion of the gene for another non-receptor tyrosine kinase, *abl*, with another gene known as *bcr* [23]. This creates a novel chimaeric protein with distinctive enzymatic and transforming properties. Because of their association with human cancer, several of the enzymes mentioned in this paragraph are among those which have been most extensively studied in the development of tyrosine kinase inhibitors.

In addition to the association of increased expression and activity of protein tyrosine kinases with various human tumours, proof of principle that these enzymes represent viable targets for cancer drug disovery is provided by the inhibitory effects of antibodies and antisense RNA together with molecular genetic experiments. Thus when recombinant DNA techniques are used to inactivate the kinase activity of either growth factor receptor-associated tyrosine kinases or src-like enzymes, the proliferative/transforming/tumorigenic capability is simultaneously eliminated [24,25].

It seems reasonable to conclude from this that inhibition of the kinase by a drug would have the same effect, although the extent to which the transphosphorylation activity must be depressed in the cells to prevent growth is unclear and remains to be elucidated.

The Issue of Selectivity

The participation of tyrosine kinases in numerous signalling pathways in normal cells clearly raises concern about the potential toxicity of such therapies. However, selectivity might be envisaged to arise by a variety of means. Tumour cells might be unusually dependent upon tyrosine phosphorylation for their proliferation. A more convincing and common view is that tyrosine kinase inhibitors could be developed with a high degree of molecular specificity for one or a few individual tyrosine kinases upon which a particular tumour type may rely heavily for proliferation/transformation signals.

A high degree of antitumour selectivity could also arise from the known degeneracy of signalling in normal cells, i.e., the existence of alternative or parallel transduction pathways which would protect the non-malignant tissue from the signalling blockade. In support of this concept, gene knock-out experiments have shown that mice deprived of certain individual non-receptor tyrosine kinases exhibit either no abnormality (*yes* and *fyn* genes), or osteoporosis due to defective osteoclast function (*src* gene), whereas double mutants for the *src/yes* or *src/fyn* genes died shortly after birth [26]. This indicates that various *src* gene family members can substitute for each other with respect to tyrosine kinase signalling in normal cells.

Nevertheless, the potential side-effects associated with inhibition of tyrosine kinases remains a concern, particularly as therapy would likely be long-term, as with, for example, tamoxifen in breast cancer. Experience will show what degree of specificity is required for an optimal balance of efficacy versus toxicity.

Screening and Design as Discovery Strategies

The considerable progress which has been made in the development of protein tyrosine kinase inhibitors has resulted from both high throughput screening and rational design approaches, and has involved natural product leads as well as synthetic medicinal chemistry applications [7-13]. In addition, knowledge of the predicted sequence of the 250-300 amino acid catalytic domain [27] coupled with the recent X-ray crystal structures of the serine/threonine kinases cAMP-dependent protein kinase (PKA, murine and porcine) [28-30] and cyclin-dependent kinase 2 (CDK2, human) [31], allows homology modelling of protein tyrosine kinases and provides insights into the reaction mechanism [32]. In practice both screening and rational design approaches are often combined as complementary elements of an iterative discovery and optimisation process.

In the EGF receptor tyrosine kinase, a conserved arginine in the catalytic loop appears to interact with the γ-phosphate of ATP; in addition, a second loop generates a binding surface that positions the phenolic hydroxyl of the tyrosine for phosphotransfer while a positively charged surface contributes to substrate recognition [32]. This greatly facilitates the computer-aided molecular design of inhibitors. While the extent to which it is desirable or possible to achieve a "clean" inhibitor of a single tyrosine kinase as opposed to a "dirtier" inhibitor of several kinase enzymes remains to be determined, it is clear that a surprising degree of molecular specificity can be obtained.

In terms of the model systems that are used in the evaluation of tyrosine kinase inhibitors, whereas natural product leads were often detected in conventional cytotoxicity screens, most groups searching for kinase inhibitors now use specially selected cell lines under

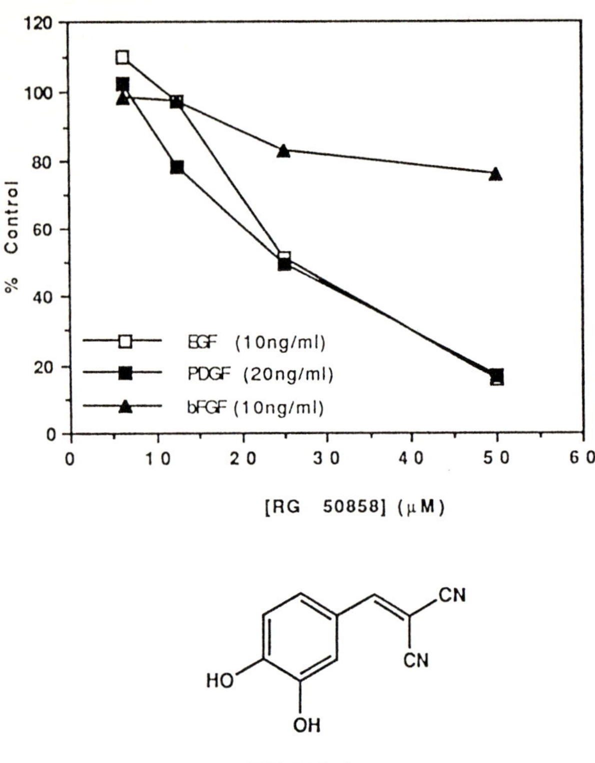

Fig. 2. Inhibition by tyrphostin RG 50858 of the growth of human glioblastoma cells stimulated by EGF, PDGF or basic FGF. Data from Brunton and Workman (unpublished).

conditions where proliferation is known to be driven by the appropriate growth factor or oncogene. In many instances enzyme assays are used as the primary screen with cell-based assays to follow. An increasing number of kinases are now being cloned and sequenced. Pharmaceutical companies in particular are in a position to screen their collections of synthetic chemicals or libraries of natural products with the aid of high throughput robotic assays. These can operate at thousands of compounds a week, using enzyme assays based on recombinant kinase domains. On the other hand, membranes from A431 squamous cell carcinomas cells have been used as a rich source of EGF receptor tyrosine kinase for drug testing [33]. Lines transfected with the appropriate kinase gene have also been employed for cell-based assays, the advantage being that direct comparison can be made with untransfected control lines. With respect to *in vivo* evaluation, human tumour xenografts expressing the appropriate growth factor receptor or

oncogene often represent the method of choice [33]. The ability to obtain evidence of enzyme inhibition within cultured cells or tumours *in vivo* is very valuable.

Table 1 illustrates some of the methodologies used for the measurement of protein tyrosine kinase activity and the effects of inhibitors.

Figure 2 shows an example from our own work in which the tyrphostin RG 50858 was found to inhibit the growth factor-dependent proliferation of a human glioblastoma cell line. This cell line responds positively to EGF, PDGF and basic FGF. It can be seen that while proliferation induced by all 3 growth factors can be inhibited by the tyrphostin, the responses to EGF and PDGF are more effectively blocked than is the stimulation by FGF. This demonstrates that selectivity for different tyrosine kinases can be more relative than absolute, which may be a desirable feature in tumours where growth is driven by multiple factors.

Chemistry of Tyrosine Kinase Inhibitors

Chemical diversity is crucial to innovative drug discovery. References 7-13 provide details on the wide variety of chemical structures identified as active against tyrosine kinases. The intention here is not to provide an exhaustive review, but rather to illustrate the background, different approaches and recent progress using selected examples.

Among the natural products, the flavonoid compounds like genistein and quercetin (Fig. 3) were important in demonstrating that inhibitors competing with ATP could nevertheless exhibit selectivity, e.g. for tyrosine kinases versus serine/threonine kinases [34]. However, the antiproliferative effects of these agents are likely to be due at least in part to their inhibition of topoisomerases [35]. Other flavonoids, such as structure c in Figure 3, are potent and selective inhibitors of the lck tyrosine kinase [36] or block tyrosine phosphorylation of the p34cdc2-type cell kinase [37]. Interestingly, the structurally related plant product piceatannol (Fig. 4) can be competitive with peptide substrate rather than ATP [38]. In a series of substituted flavones, 3'-amino-4'-methoxyflavone was the most cytotoxic against fibroblasts transformed with *abl*, with some selectivity versus the non-transformed cells; however, although this agent

Table 1. Methodology for measurement of protein tyrosine kinase activity

Protein tyrosine kinase	Substrate	Source
In vitro measurement of protein tyrosine kinase activity		
EGFR	autophosphorylation angiotensin II poly(GAT) RR-SRC peptide	A431 cells: human squamous carcinoma
EGFRIC	PLCAγ-1254 peptide	Purified intracellular domain EGFR from A431 cells
PDGFR	autophosphorylation	NIH 3T3 cells: normal mouse fibroblasts
p185^{erbB2}	autophosphorylation	TMK-1 cells: human gastric carcinoma
	autophosphorylation	NIH 3T3 cells transfected with HER1-2 chimaeric protein:ligand binding domain of erbB2 replaced with EGF binding domain of EGFR
Insulin RK	poly(GAT)	Placenta, liver
pp60^{src}	autophosporylation enolase α-casein	RSV-transformed NIH 3T3 cells
	autophosphorylation α-casein	tsNRK cells: normal rat kidney cells transformed with T class mutant RSV
	autophosphorylation calpactin I	RR 1022 cells: newborn rat tumour line transformed by RSV
	autophosporylation enolase	TMK-1 cells
	poly(GT)	RSV transformed quail cells
p56^{lck}	autophosphorylation enolase angiotensin I	Bovine thymus
	autophosphorylation angiotensin I	LSTRA cells
p210$^{bcr-abl}$	autophosphorylation poly(GAT)	K562 ? human myeloid leukaemia
p60^{v-abl}	angiotensin II α-casein	Recombinant v-abl expressed in E. coli
In situ measurement of protein tyrosine kinase activity		
EGFR		A431 cells HER14 cells: NIH 3T3 cells transfected with EGFR
PDGFR		Vascular smooth muscle cells

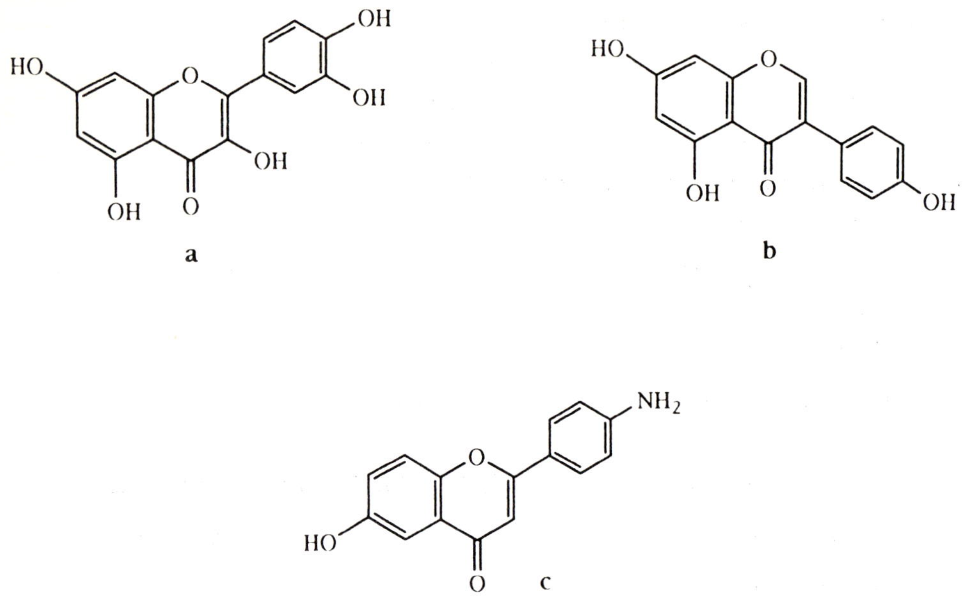

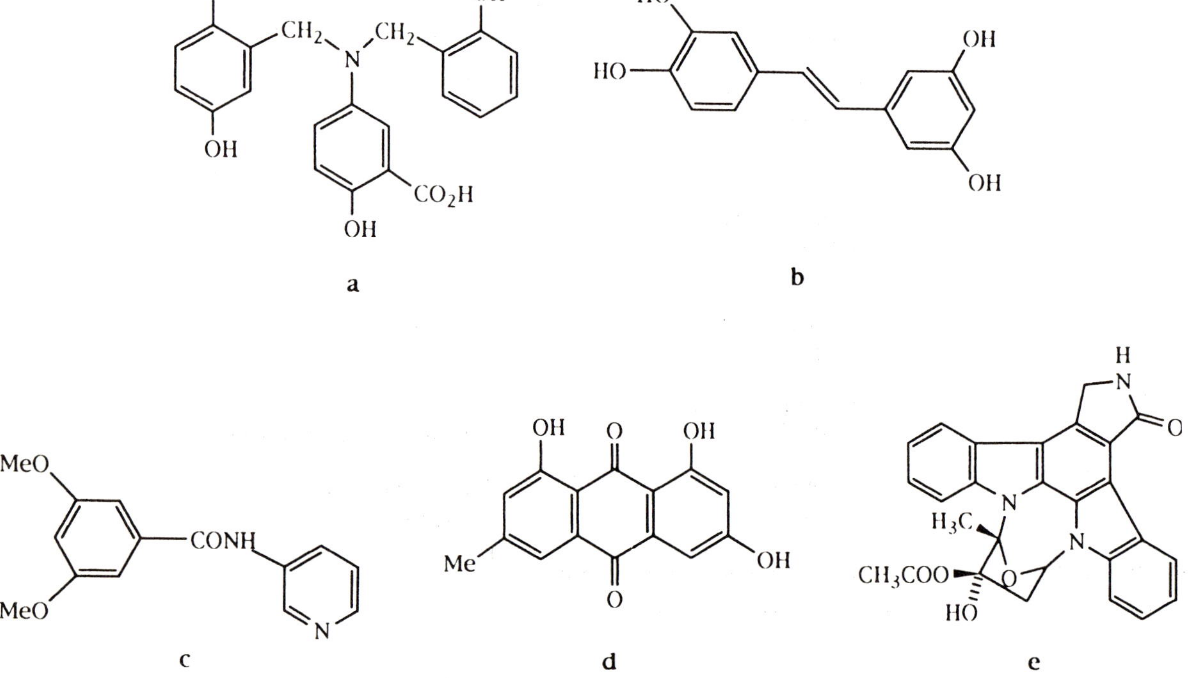

Fig. 3. Structures of flavonoid tyrosine kinase inhibitors: quercetin (a), genistein (b) and an amino flavonoid analogue (c). See text and reference 10 for more details.

Fig. 4. Structures of a range of mainly natural product tyrosine kinase inhibitors: lavendustin A (a), piceatannol (b), one of a series of stilbene and amide derivatives based on piceatannol (c), emodin (d) and the staurosporin-related agent K252a (e). See text and reference 10 for more details.

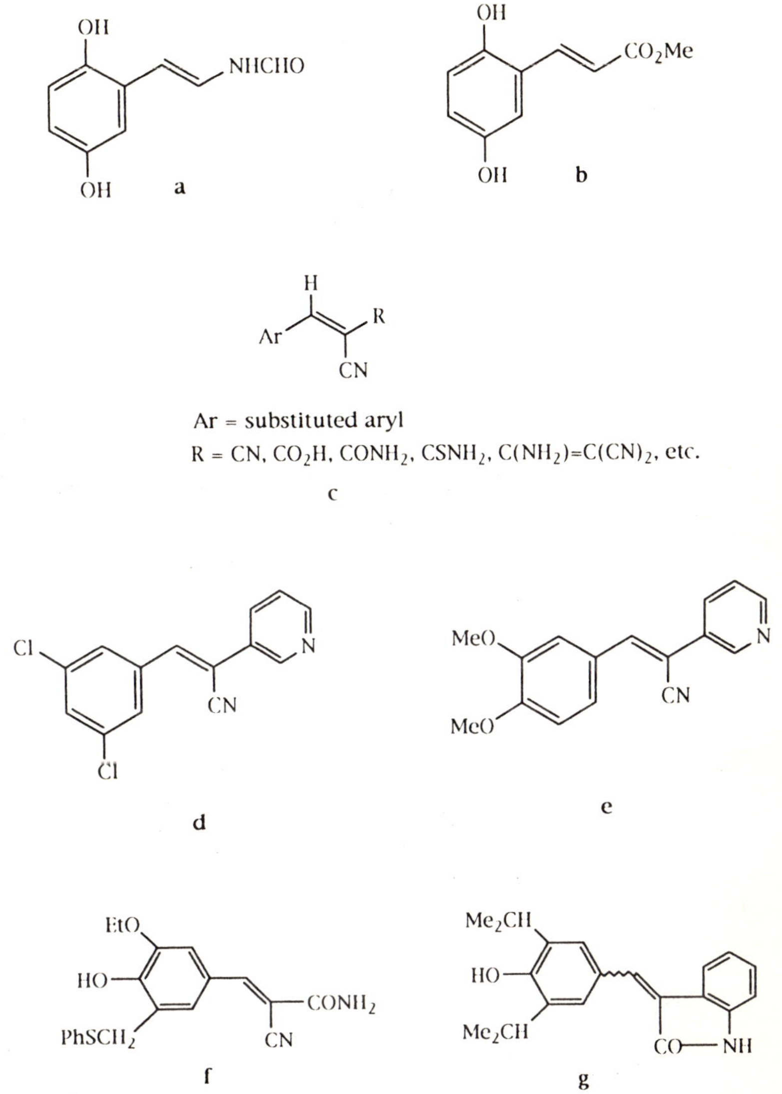

Fig. 5. Structures of erbstatin (a) and related compounds: 2,5 dihydroxycinnamate (b), tyrphostins (c) such as RG 14620 (d) and RG 13022 (e), and α-cyanocinnamide derivatives ST 280 (f) and ST 638 (g). See text and reference 10 for further details.

inhibited the EGF receptor kinase, it was inactive against the *abl*-encoded kinase [39].

Demonstration of tyrosine kinase inhibition and antitumour activity of the styrene-containing natural product erbstatin [40] (Fig. 5) led to the impressive benzylidene malanonitrile analogues known as tyrphostins [8]. Of particular interest is the reported ability to discriminate not only between tyrosine versus serine/threonine kinases, but also between individual tyrosine kinases, e.g. EGF versus insulin receptor kinases [41] and even the closely related EGF versus erbB2/neu receptor enzymes [42]. Tyrphostins are competitive with protein substrate and may be competitive or noncompetitive with ATP. Structure-activity relationships demonstrated the importance of planarity and hydroxylation in the molecule. In our own work we have confirmed and extended the observation that inhibitory potency is enhanced by increasing ring hydroxylation; however, in an attempt to avoid this potentially adverse structural feature from a stability and drug metabolism point of view, we found that heteroaromatic replacements were generally less active on the EGF receptor enzyme while still inhibiting growth factor-induced proliferation, possibly via inhibition of other kinases [43]. A further significant development was the demonstration of *in vitro* and *in vivo* antitumour activity with potentially more stable second generation tyrphostin derivatives lacking hydroxyl substituents [44]. Additional tyrosine mimics with good inhibitory activity include hydroxycinnamides [45] and nitrostyrenes [46].

In relation to the latter, a very interesting approach has involved the synthesis of potential bisubstrate or transition state analogues featur-

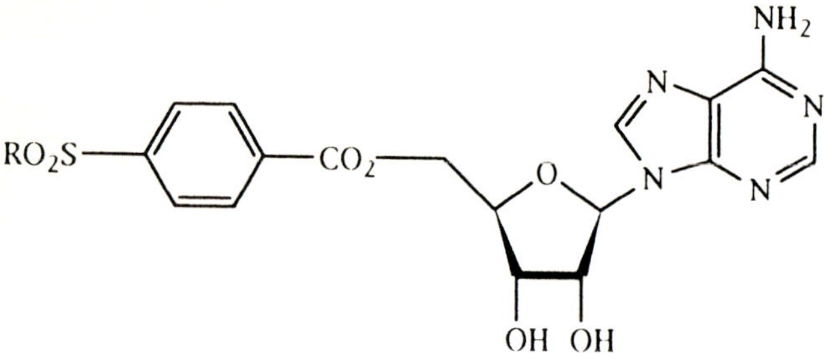

a R = F
b R = NHPh

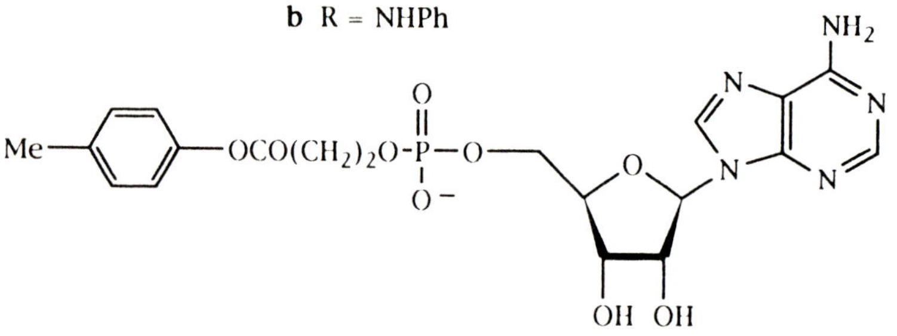

c

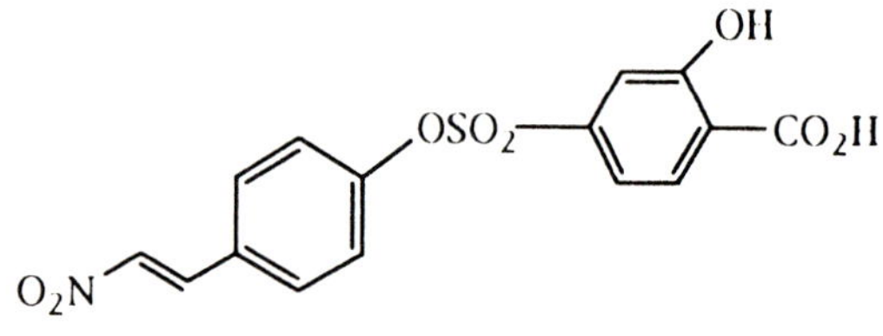

d

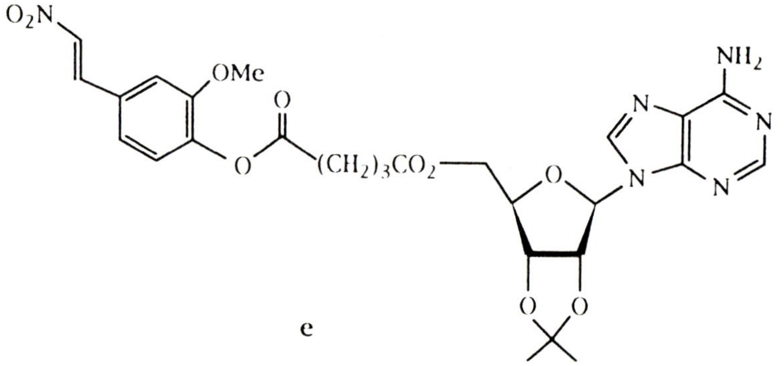

e

Fig. 6. Structures of multisubstrate tyrosine kinase inhibitors including the sulphonamide derivative (b) of the ATP analogue FSBA (a), a related transition state analogue (c), a compound incorporating the sulphonylbenzyl moiety of FSBA linked to a nitrostyrene (d), and an analogue replacing the sulphonylbenzyl moiety with glutaric acid (e). See text and reference 10 for further details.

ing a tyrosine mimic in combination with an ATP cofactor mimic or spacer, as for example with the sulfonylbenzoyl-nitrostyrenes (Fig. 6), which were potent and selective inhibitors of the EGF receptor kinase [46]. Other potent and selective tyrosine kinase inhibitors were provided by the thiazolidine-diones [47], amino-alkyl-acrylophenones [48] and thioindoles [49]. Surprisingly, whereas the natural product staurosporine was unselective across tyrosine and serine/threonine kinases and certain agly-

cone analogues are highly specific for protein kinase C, a novel series of related dianilinophthalimides have proved recently to be highly active against the EGF-receptor tyrosine kinase but inactive on protein kinase C [50,51]. Such agents not only exhibit potent antiproliferative activity *in vitro*, but also display promising antitumour efficacy *in vivo* at well tolerated doses [51].

A further series of tyrosine kinase inhibitors which show significant antitumour activity *in*

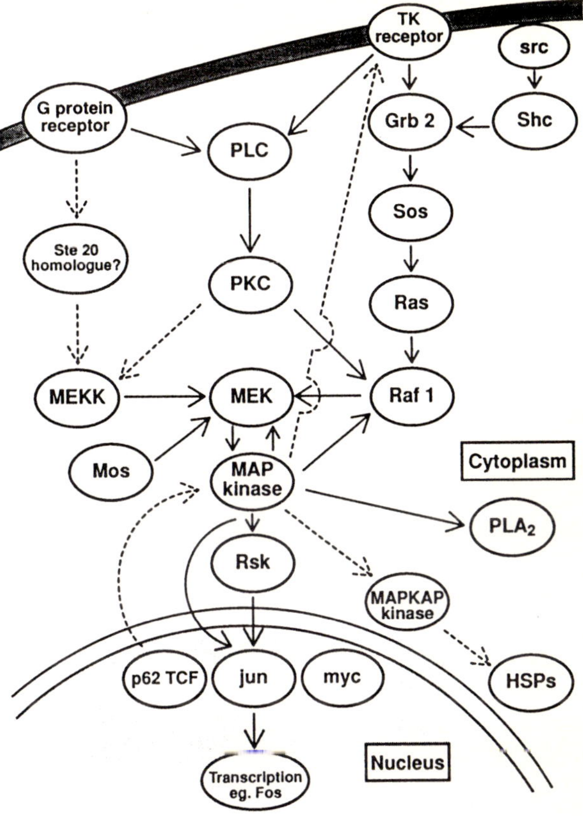

Fig. 8. Convergent MAP kinase activation pathways. MAP kinase is activated by MAP kinase kinase, also known as MEK, which is in turn activated either: 1) by the MAP kinase kinase kinase or MEK kinase raf 1 via the receptor tyrosine kinase-ras pathway, also used by src; or 2) by the alternative MAP kinase kinase kinase or MEK kinase known as MEKK, which is activated through both heptahelical membrane G protein-linked and membrane tyrosine kinase-linked receptors via PLC and PKC (and possibly other mechanisms such as a mammalian homologue of the yeast Ste 20). The oncogene product mos also activates MEK. In addition to activating nuclear transcription factors directly and/or via rsk, MAP kinase also phosphorylates MEK, EGF receptor, PLA$_2$ and MAPKAP kinase which in turn phosphorylates the 25kD and 27kD heat shock proteins. Solid arrows indicate interactions which are strongly defined, while dotted arrows indicate less definite links. For further details see text and references 55-57.

Fig. 7. Structure of the benzoquinoid ansamycin, herbimycin A. See text and reference 10 for further details.

vivo are the benzoquinoid ansamycin antibiotics typified by herbimycin A (Fig. 7) and geldanamycin [52]. These agents inhibit the src tyrosine kinase among others, and this has been correlated with reversion of src transformation [52]. Abolition of inhibitory activity by thiol reagents suggests a mechanism involving sulphydryls in the kinase [53]. Other recent work suggests that herbimycin A inhibits the association of p60 v-src with the cytoskeleton and with an important downstream effector, phosphatidylinositol 3'kinase (PI3 kinase) [54]. A potential problem with such quinone-containing agents is the complications introduced by metabolic redox cycling leading to oxidative stress and DNA damage.

Signalling Downstream of Tyrosine Kinases: Mechanisms and Targets

What is the mechanism by which tyrosine phosphorylation leads to cell proliferation? Over the last year, essentially all of the key players involved in the mitogenic signal transduction cascade linking growth factor receptors on the cell membrane through the G-protein ras to the activation of transcription factors and the consequent expression of early response genes (such as *fos*) have been identified [55,56]. The essential features are shown in Figures 8 and 9. Ligand docking and the consequent autophosphorylation of intrinsic tyrosine kinase receptors leads to binding to the cytosolic domain of the receptors via their so-called SH2 domains (which recognise specific

phosphotyrosine-containing peptide sequences) of various effector molecules such as PI3 kinase and phospholipase C γ and also of certain adaptor molecules such as grb2 [57]. These specific interactions between SH2 domains and particular phosphotyrosine residues can be blocked by the corresponding phosphorylated peptide sequence [58,59]. Grb2 binds the guanine nucleotide exchange factor sos via SH3 domain interaction and recruits it to

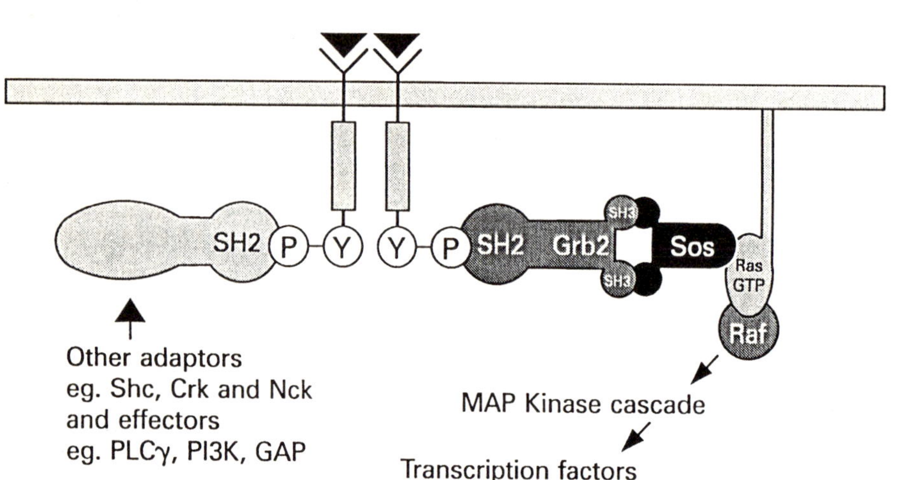

Fig. 9. A more detailed view of signal transduction through protein tyrosine kinase receptors. On the right, the grb2 adaptor protein is shown to bind to a specific phosphotyrosine residue on the receptor via its src homology 2 (SH2) domain. This in turn is coupled to the sos guanine nucleotide exchange factor via its SH3 domains, thereby converting ras to the GTP-bound form. Ras then activates the serine/threonine kinase cascade involving sequentially raf 1 which acts as a MAP kinase kinase kinase, MAP kinase kinase (also known as MEK) and MAP kinase itself, with input also possible via protein kinase C. MAP kinase translocates to the nucleus where it phosphorylates transcription factors, such as myc and jun, and also the pp62 ternary complex factor, which binds to the serum response element leading to *fos* expression. Another potentially important serine/threonine kinase is pp90 RSK which is a substrate for MAP kinase and also translocates to the nucleus. On the left are shown other adaptors (e.g. shc, crk and nck) and effectors (e.g. phospholipase Cγ, phosphatidylinositol 3'kinase and rasGAP) which also bind to specific phosphotyrosines on the receptor via their SH2 domains. Modified from reference 60. For further details see text and references 56 and 57.

the cell membrane where it converts ras from the inactive GDP-bound form to the GTP-bound active conformation. In turn, ras binds and activates the serine/threonine kinase raf, probably with the involvement of an additional kinase. Next, raf phosphorylates another kinase called MEK and this then phosphorylates MAP kinase on both serine and tyrosine. Following this unusual activation event, MAP kinase phosphorylates and activates a number of key signalling proteins including another protein kinase, rsk, phospholipase A2 and, importantly, certain transcription factors such as p62TCF, myc and jun, leading to gene expression.

The central importance of the ras-raf-MAP kinase cascade to signal transduction is underlined by the demonstration that various other oncogenes and signalling proteins also feed into key points of the pathway. Thus src binds grb2 via shc, heptahelical G-protein-linked receptors activate MEK via the raf homologue MEKK, and mos also activates MEK. Furthermore, the growth inhibitory pathway involving cyclic AMP and protein kinase C functions by inhibiting signal transduction between ras and raf, apparently via direct phosphorylation of raf by protein kinase A or alternatively via the protein rap 1 which acts as a competitive inhibitor of ras [61-63].

Extensive "cross-talk" is a feature of various interconnected signal transduction pathways. While the MAP kinases are emerging as crucial signal integrator molecules, the extensive family of protein kinase C isoenzymes are also seen as critical intermediaries between various transduction highways. Importantly, the different protein kinase C isoforms not only exhibit distinct patterns of tissue-specific expression, they also display disparate activation patterns with respect to activation by numerous products of lipid signalling cascades.

It should also be noted that there is a more direct, ras-independent growth factor signalling pathway involving tyrosine phosphorylation of transcription factors p91 and SIF-A [64-66]. The significance of this remains to be established. Of course, the potentially branched rather than linear nature may present problems in terms of their blockade by drugs. But in addition to providing escape routes for resistance mechanisms, the presence of distinct wiring diagrams in different cell types also provides potential options for therapeutic selectivity.

The elucidation of the major signalling trunk route involving tyrosine kinase → ras → raf → MAP kinase cascade has important implications

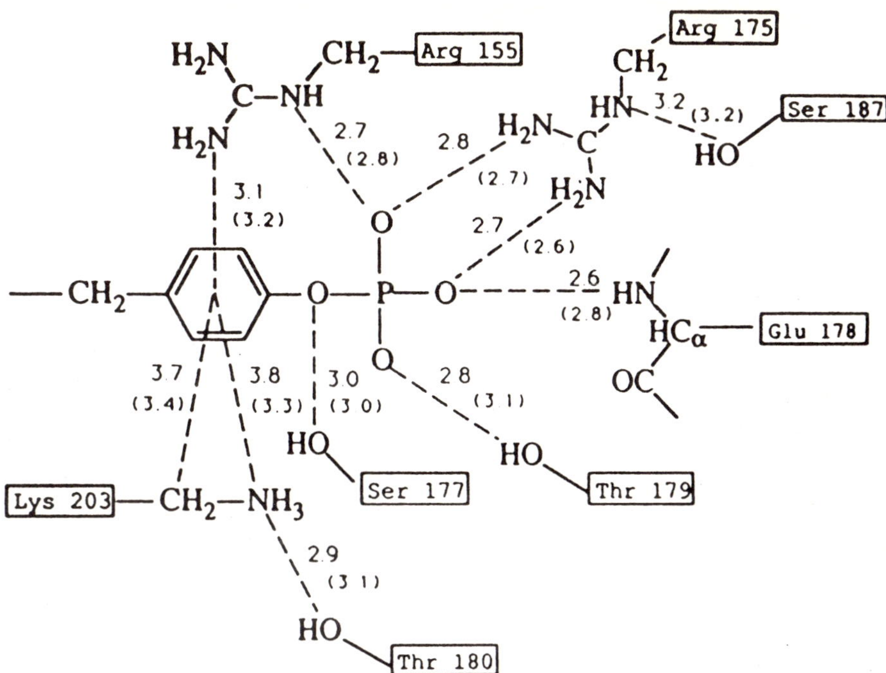

Fig. 10. Schematic diagram of the specific phosphotyrosine SH2 recognition domain of v-src complexed to a phosphotyrosyl peptide. The X-ray crystal structure shows that a central antiparallel ß-sheet in the SH2 domain is flanked by a pair of α-helices. The molecular recognition involves amino-aromatic interactions between lysine and arginine side chains of the protein with the tyrosine ring system in addition to the hydrogen bonding with the phosphate. Reproduced with permission from reference 70.

for the potential utility of tyrosine kinase inhibitors in cancer and for the selection of alternative molecular targets for drug discovery. Reference to Figure 8 will reveal that if the tyrosine kinase cascade is activated downstream of the kinase, for example at ras or raf, then it is unlikely that a specific inhibitor of an upstream kinase would be effective. Further inspection of Figure 8 will, however, allow numerous alternative targets to be selected for the therapy of such tumours: for example, it is clear that in such a situation a specific inhibitor of MAP kinase would be active although a possible downside (or advantage?) is that a wider range of pathways would be blocked.

Ras gene mutations which are very common in human cancers cause the ras molecular switch to be continually "jammed on" [67]. An exciting new development therefore has been the demonstration of selective inhibition of the proliferation/transformation of cells containing mutant oncogenic *ras* genes by peptide mimetics that inhibit the farnesylation reaction which is essential for membrane docking and signal transduction [68,69]. The next phase will be to achieve *in vivo* antitumour activity using this approach.

The possibility of selective antagonism of particular SH2 domain-phosphotyrosine docking interactions as a means of blocking signal transduction has now gained prominence with the demonstration that specific phosphotyrosine-containing peptides can display inhibitory activity [58,59]. Structural elucidation of phosphopeptide-SH2 binding mechanisms by X-ray crystallography and nuclear magnetic resonance spectroscopy should greatly facilitate this approach [70]. Figure 10 illustrates how for the binding of the SH2 domain of v-src with a phosphotyrosyl peptide this involves interactions between lysine and arginine side chains of the protein with the aromatic tyrosine, together with hydrogen bonding to the phosphate.

The development of agents capable of selectively inhibiting tyrosine kinase, ras and other key points on the signalling cascade shown in Figure 8 should allow us to identify which targets are most appropriate to generate selective antitumour efficacy. It is quite possible that this may vary according to the oncogene/signal transduction profile of particular tumours.

The Cytostatic versus Cytotoxic Issue

We can envisage inhibitors of oncogenic tyrosine kinases and other drugs acting on signal transduction targets like ras as a logical extension of the classical antihormonal agents, e.g. tamoxifen. We might therefore anticipate a scenario in which such inhibitors would be given

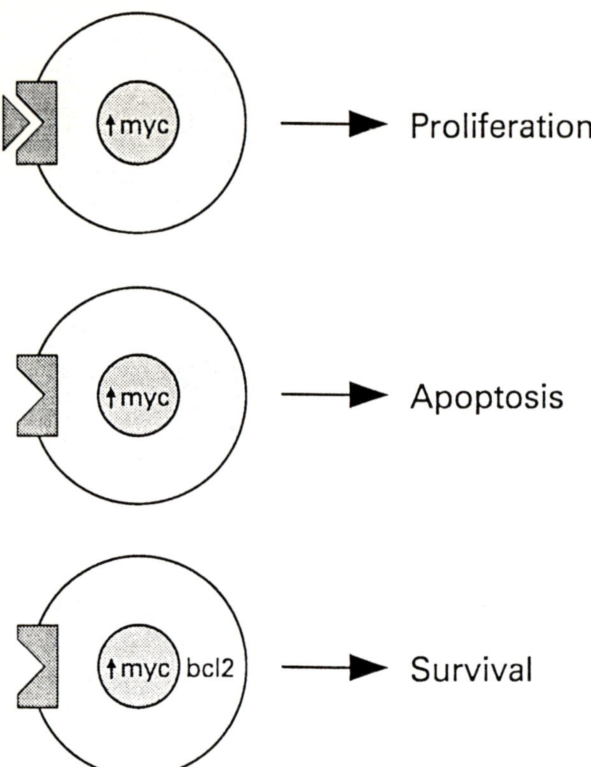

Fig. 11. The interactions of growth factors, deregulated *myc* gene expression and the *bcl2* oncogene product in controlling proliferation, apoptosis and survival. When the *myc* gene is hyperexpressed and tyrosine kinase growth factor receptors are activated by ligand, a proliferative response is seen (top). If the growth factor is removed, apoptosis or programmed cell death occurs (middle). However, if growth factor is removed from a cell with hyperexpressed *myc* gene and also the *bcl2* gene expressed, survival without proliferation is seen. Other growth stimulating signals could substitute for tyrosine kinase receptor stimulation (e.g. ras or raf activation) and alternative survival genes or loss of tumour suppressor genes (e.g. *p53*) could contribute to survival in a complex network of interactions. In the model shown, inhibition of the receptor tyrosine kinase or a downstream signal might be expected to have the same effect as removal of growth factor, i.e. apoptosis (middle panel).

chronically to suppress growth over a prolonged period. Hence a relatively clean side-effect profile is necessary. According to this simple model this type of antisignalling agent would be cytostatic rather than cytotoxic.

Such an outcome would be quite acceptable in therapeutic terms in that, although cell killing might not occur, tumour growth would still be blocked. However, the results emerging from the exciting arena of programmed cell death or apoptosis (see refs. 71-74 and the chapter by

Bursch in this volume) suggest that this may not necessarily be the case. Of particular importance is the fact that in cells with deregulated oncogenes such as *myc* (typically most tumours), whereas the addition of growth factors stimulates proliferation, removal of the growth factors causes *myc* gene expression to induce apoptosis [75]. If, however, the cell also expresses the *bcl2* "survival" oncogene, removal of growth factors does not lead to apoptosis. This is depicted schematically in Figure 11. With respect to tyrosine kinase inhibitors, this model would predict that blockade of the kinase cascade would be equivalent to removal of growth factors. Thus in a cell with deregulated *myc* but lacking *bcl2* expression cell death might ensue, whereas in the simultaneous presence of *bcl2* expression, cytostasis but survival would be seen. At the moment, however, there appears to be no clear pharmacological evidence on this issue, which might well impact on how a tyrosine kinase blocker was used clinically.

Concluding Remarks

As tyrosine kinase inhibitors move steadily towards the clinic, it is essential that their special properties as signal transduction cancer drugs are understood and acted upon. Preclinical models used for testing (see also the chapter by D'Incalci in this volume) and patients to be treated should both be selected on the basis of known involvement of an oncogenic tyrosine kinase. Conventional administration schedules and maximum tolerated doses are unlikely to be appropriate. Optimisation of pharmacokinetics to provide sustained enzyme inhibition will be necessary for success [76]. Having pharmacodynamic assays in place which provide data on biochemical as well as gross therapeutic responses, will also be very important.

This discussion has mainly focused on the inhibition of tyrosine kinases known to be involved in cell proliferation. However, the focal adhesion kinase (p125FAK) has been proposed to function at a point of convergence in the action of oncogenes, neuropeptides and integrins [77] and may play a key role in invasion [78]. Interestingly, there is increasingly strong evidence that the tyrosine kinase receptor for vascular endothelial growth factor (VEGF) is a major contributor to angiogenesis [79].

An optimistic view would be that tyrosine kinase inhibitors will be only the first of many effective "designer" drugs fashioned to combat specific oncogenic changes in cancer cells. Complementary to antisense and gene therapy approaches, blockade of signal transduction provides the exciting prospect of a portfolio of highly selective therapies which can be targeted specifically to the particular genetic and biochemical make-up of an individual patient's tumour. Bespoke gene therapy and signal transduction modulation may not be so futuristic as it may at first seem, and tyrosine kinase inhibitors are well positioned to be in the vanguard of the new cancer pharmacology.

Acknowledgements

We are grateful to the Cancer Research Campaign (CRC) for financial support. Paul Workman acknowledges the award of a CRC Life Fellowship.

REFERENCES

1   Johnson RK: Screening methods in drug discovery. JNCI 1990 (82):1082-1083
2   Schwartsmann G and Workman P: Anticancer drug screening and discovery in the 1990s: A European perspective. Eur J Cancer 1993 (29A):3-14
3   Workman P (ed) New anticancer drug design based on advances in molecular oncology. Sem Cancer Biol 1992 (3):329-333
4   Vogelstein B and Kinzler KW: The multistep nature of cancer. Trends Genetics 1993 (9):138-141
5   Powis G: Signalling targets for anticancer drug development. Trends Pharm Sci 1991 (12):188-193
6   Brunton VG and Workman P: Cell-signalling targets for antitumour drug development. Cancer Chemother Pharmacol 1993 (32):1-19
7   Kenyon GL and Garcia GA: Design of kinase inhibitors. Med Res Rev 1987 (7):389-416
8   Levitski A: Tyrphostins - potential antiproliferative agents and novel molecular tools. Biochem Pharmac 1990 (40):313-318
9   Chang C-J and Geahlen RL: Protein-tyrosine kinase inhibition: mechanism-based discovery of antitumor agents. J Natural Products 1992 (11):1529-1560
10 Workman P, Brunton VG, Robins DJ: Tyrosine kinase inhibitors. Sem Cancer Biol 1992 (3):369-381
11 Burke TR: Protein-tyrosine kinase inhibitors. Drugs of the Future 1992 (17):119-131
12 Spence P: Inhibitors of tyrosine kinase activity as anticancer therapeutics: recent developments. Current Opinion in Therapeutic Patents, December 1992
13 Dobrusin EM and Fry DW: Protein tyrosine kinases and cancer. Ann Rep Med Chem 1992 (27):169-176
14 Hunter T: A thousand and one protein kinases. Cell 1987 (50):823-829
15 Gescher A: Towards selective pharmacological modulation of protein kinase C - opportunities for the development of novel antineoplastic agents. Br J Cancer 1992 (66):10-19
16 Grunicke HH and Uberall F: Protein kinase C modulation. Sem Cancer Biology 1992 (3):351-360
17 Fantl W, Johnson DE, Williams RT: Signalling by receptor tyrosine kinases. Ann Rev Biochem 1993 (62):453-481
18 Slamon DJ, Clark GM, Wong SG, Levin WJ, Ullrich A, McGuire WL: Human breast cancer: correlation of relapse and survival with amplification of the HER-2/*neu* oncogene. Science 1987 (235):177-181
19 Slamon DJ, Godolphin W, Jones LA et al: Studies of HER-2/*neu* proto-oncogene in human breast and ovarian cancer. Science 1989 (244):707-712
20 Bicknell R and Harris AL: Anticancer strategies involving vasculature: vascular targeting and the inhibition of angiogenesis. Sem Cancer Biology 1992 (3):399-407
21 Bolen JB, Veillette A, Schwartz A, DeSeau V, Rosen N: Activation of pp60^{c-src} protein kinase activity in human colon carcinoma. Proc Natl Acad Sci 1987 (84):2251-2255
22 Ottenhoff-Kalff AE, Rijksen G, van Bearden EACM, Hennipman A, Michels AA, Staal GEJ: Characterization of protein tyrosine kinases from human breast cancer: Involvement of the c-src oncogene product. Cancer Res 1992 (52):4773-4778
23 Shtivelman E, Lifshitz B, Gale RP, Canaani E: Fused transcript of *abl* and *bcr* genes in chronic myelogenous leukaemia. Nature 1985 (315):550-554
24 Ullrich A and Schlessinger J: Signal transduction by receptors with tyrosine kinase activity. Cell 1990 (61):203-213
25 Snyder MA, Bishop JM, McGrath JP, Levinson AD: A mutation at the ATP-binding site of pp60^{c-src} abolishes kinase activity, transformation, and tumorigenicity. Mol Cell Biol 1985 (5):1772-1779
26 Stein PL, Imamoto A, Soriano P: Genetic analysis of *src*-family tyrosine kinase mouse mutants. Proc Am Assoc Cancer Res 1993 (34):575
27 Hanks SK, Quinn AM, Hunter T: The protein kinase family: conserved features and deduced phylogeny of the catalytic domains. Science 1988 (241):42-52
28 Knighton DR, Zheng J, Ten Eyck LF, Ashford VA, Xuong N-H, Taylor SS, Sowadski JM: Crystal structure of the catalytic subunit of cyclic adenosine monophosphate-dependent protein kinase. Science 1991 (253):407-414
29 Zheng J, Knighton DR, Ten Eyck LF, Karlsson R, Xuong N-H, Taylor S, Sowadski JM: Crystal structure of the catalytic subunit of cAMP-dependent protein kinase complexed with MgATP and peptide inhibitor. Biochemistry 1993 (32):2154-2161
30 Bossemeyer D, Engh RA, Kinzel V, Ponstinyl H, Huber R: Phosphotransferase and substrate binding mechanism of the cAMP-dependent protein kinase catalytic subunit from porcine heart as deduced from the 2.0 Å structure of the complex with Mn^{2+} adenyl imidophosphate and inhibitor peptide PKI (5-24). EMBO J 1993 (3):849-859
31 De Bondt HL, Rosenblatt J, Jancarik J, Jones HD, Morgan DO, Kim S-H: Crystal structure of cyclin-dependent kinase 2. Science 1993 (363):595-603
32 Knighton DR, Cadena DL, Zheng J, Ten Eyck LF, Taylor SS, Sowadski JM, Gill GN: Structural features that specify tyrosine kinase activity deduced from homology modelling of the epidermal growth factor receptor. Proc Natl Acad Sci 1993 (90):5001-5005
33 Robinson S, Dean BJ, Petty BA: Characterization of A431 tumor xenograft as an in vivo model for testing epidermal growth factor-receptor antagonists. Int J Oncol 1992 (1):293-298
34 Hagiwara M, Inoue S, Tanaka T, Nunoki K, Ito M, Hidaka H: Differential effects of flavonoids as inhibitors of tyrosine protein kinases and serine/threonine protein kinases. Biochem Pharmac 1988 (37):2987-2992
35 Okura A, Arakawa H, Oka H, Yoshinari T, Moden Y: Effect of genistein on topoisomerase activity and on the growth of Ha-*ras*-transformed NIH3T3 cells. Biochem Biophys Res Comm 1988 (157):183-189
36 Cushman M, Nagarathnam D, Burg DL, Geahlen RL: Synthesis and protein tyrosine kinase inhibitory activities of flavonoid analogues. J Med Chem 1991 (34):798-806
37 Worland PJ, Kaur G, Stetler-Stevenson M, Sebers S, Sartor O, Sausville EA: Alteration of a p34^{cdc2}

kinase by the flavone L86-8275 in breast carcinoma cells. Biochem Pharmac 1993 (46):1831-1840

38 Geahlen RL and McLaughlin JL: Piceatannol (3,4,5'-tetrahydroxy-*trans*-stilbene) is a naturally occurring protein-tyrosine kinase inhibitor. Biochem Biophys Res Comm 1989 (165):241-245

39 Cunningham BDM, Threadgill MD, Groundwater PW, Dale IL, Hickman JA: Synthesis and biological evaluation of protein tyrosine kinases. Anti-Cancer Drug Design 1992 (7):365-384

40 Umezawa H, Imoto M, Sawa T, Isshiki K, Matsuda N, Uchida T, Iinuma H, Hamada H, Hamada M, Takeuchi T: Studies on a new epidermal growth factor receptor kinase inhibitor, erbstatin, produced by MH 435-hF3. J Antibiot 1986 (39):170-173

41 Yaish P, Gazit A, Gilon C, Levitski A: Blocking of EGF-dependent cell proliferation by EGF receptor kinase inhibitors. Science 1988 (242):933-935

42 Gazit A, Osherov N, Posner I, Yaish P, Pradosy E, Gilon C, Levitski A: Tyrphostins 2. Heterocyclic and alpha-substituted benzylidenemalononitrile tyrphostins as potent inhibitors of EGF receptor and erbB2/neu tyrosine kinases. J Med Chem 1991 (34):1897-1907

43 Brunton VG, Lear MJ, Robins DJ, Williamson S, Workman P: Synthesis and antiproliferative activity of tyrphostins containing heteroaromatic moieties. Anti-Cancer Drug Design 1994 (in press)

44 Yoneda T, Lyall RM, Alsina MM, Persons PE, Spada AP, Levitski A, Zilbertstein A, Mundy GR: The antiproliferative effects of tyrosine kinase inhibitors tyrphostins and a human squamous cell carcinoma in vitro and in nude mice. Cancer Res 1991 (51):4430-4435

45 Shiraishi T, Domoto T, Imai N, Shimada Y, Watanabe K: Specific inhibitors of tyrosine specific protein kinase, synthetic 4-hydroxycinnamamide derivatives. Biochem Biophys Res Comm 1987 (147):322-328

46 Traxler PM, Wacker O, Bach HL, Geissler JF, Kump W, Meyer T, Regenass U, Roesel JL, Lydon N: Sulfonylbenzoylnitrostyrenes: potential bisubstrate type inhibitors of the EGF-receptor tyrosine kinase. J Med Chem 1991 (34):2328-2337

47 Geissler JF, Traxler P, Regenass U, Murray BJ, Roessel JL, Meyer T, McGlynn E, Storni A, Lydon NB: Thiazolidine-diones. Biochemical and biological activity of a novel class of tyrosine protein kinase inhibitors. J Biol Chem 1990 (265):22255-22261

48 Traxler P, Buchdunger E, Mett H, Meyer T, Regenass U, Roesel J, Trinks U, Lydon N: Amino-alkyl-acrylophenones as potent and selective inhibitors of the EGF-receptor protein tyrosine kinase. Proc Am Assoc Cancer Res 1992 (33):527

49 Kraker AJ, Wemple, Schemmel ME, Moore CW: Inhibition of epidermal growth factor receptor tyrosine kinase by 2-thioindoles, a new structural class of tyrosine kinase inhibitor. Proc Am Assoc Cancer Res 1993 (34):408

50 Lydon N, Buchdunger E, Mett H, Regenass U, Muller M, Trinks U, Traxler P: Biological profile of CGP 52411: a tyrosine protein kinase inhibitor with selectivity for the EGF-receptor enzyme family. J Cell Biochem Suppl 1993 (17A):235

51 Buchdunger F et al: 4,5-dianilino-phthalimide: a novel tyrosine protein kinase inhibitor with selectivity for the EGF receptor signal transduction pathway and potent *in vivo* antitumour activity. Proc Natl Acad Sci 1994 (in press)

52 Uchara Y, Hori M, Takeuchi T, Umezawa H: Screening of agents which convert 'transformed morphology': identification of an active agent as herbimycin and its inhibition of intracellular *src* kinase. Jpn J Cancer Res 1985 (76):672-675

53 Uchara Y, Fukazawa H, Murakami Y, Mizuno S: Irreversible inhibition of v-*src* tyrosine kinase activity by herbimycin A and its abrogation by sulphydryl compounds. Biochem Biophys Res Comm 1989 (163):803-809

54 Hamaguchi M, Xiao H, Uchara Y, Ohnishi Y, Nagai Y: Herbimycin A inhibits the association of p60[v-src] with the cytoskeletal structure and with phosphatidylinositol 3'kinase. Oncogene 1993 (8):559-564

55 Pelech L: Networking with protein kinases. Current Biology 1993 (3):513-515

56 Moodie SA and Wolfman A: The 3 Rs of life: Ras, raf and growth regulation. Trends Genetics 1994 (10): 44-48

57 Pawson T and Schlessinger J: SH2 and SH3 domains. Current Biology 1993 (3):434-442

58 Songyang Z, Schoelson SE, Chaudhuri M et al: SH2 domains recognize specific phosphopeptide sequences. Cell 1993 (72):767-778

59 McNamara DJ, Dobrusin E, Zhu G, Decker SJ, Saltiel AR: Inhibition of the binding of phospholipase Cγ1 SH2 domains to phosphorylated epidermal growth factor receptor by phosphorylated peptides. Int J Peptide Protein Res 1993 (42):240-248

60 McCormick F: How receptors turn ras on. Nature 1993 (363):15-16

61 Wu J, Dent P, Jelinek T, Wolfman A, Weber M, Sturgill TW: Inhibition of the EGF-activated MAP kinase signalling pathway by adenosine 3',5'-monophosphate. Science 1993 (262):1065-1069

62 Cook SJ and McCormick F: Inhibition by cAMP of ras-dependent activation of raf. Science 1993 (262):1069-1072

63 Graves LM, Bornfeldt KE, Raines EW, Potts BC, MacDonald SG, Ross R, Krebs EG: Protein kinase A antagonizes platelet-derived growth factor-induced signalling by mitogen-activated protein kinase in human arterial smooth muscle cells. Proc Natl Acad Sci USA 1993 (90):10300-10304

64 Silvennoinen O, Schindler C, Schlessinger J, Levy DE: *Ras*-independent growth factor signalling by transcription factor tyrosine phosphorylation. Science 1993 (261):1736-1739

65 Sadowski HB, Shuai K, Darnell JE, Gilman MZ: A common nuclear signal transduction pathway activated by growth factor and cytokine receptors. Science 1993 (261):1739-1743

66 Fu X-Y and Zhang J-J: Transcription factor p91 interacts with the epidermal growth factor receptor and mediates activation of the c-*fos* gene promoter. Cell 1993 (74):1135-1145

67 Bos JL: *Ras* oncogenes and human cancer: A review. Cancer Res 1989 (49):4682-4689

68 James GL, Goldstein JL, Brown MS et al: Benzodiazepine peptidomimetics: Potent inhibitors

of ras farnesylation in animal cells. Science 1993 (260):1937-1942

69 Kohl NE, Mosser SD, de Solms J, Giuliani EA, Pompliano DL, Graham SL, Smith RL, Scolnick EM, Oliff A, Gibbs JB: Selective inhibition of *ras*-dependent transformation by a farnesyltransferase inhibitor. Science 1993 (260):1934-1937

70 Waksman G, Kominos D, Robertson SC et al: Crystal structure of the phosphotyrosine recognition domain SH2 of v-*src* complexed with tyrosine-phosphorylated peptides. Nature 1992 (358):646-653

71 Kerr JFR, Wyllie AH, Currie AR: Apoptosis: a basic biological phenomenon with wide ranging implications in tissue kinetics. Br J Cancer 1972 (26):239-157

72 Wyllie AH, Kerr JFR, Currie AR: Cell death: the significance of apoptosis. Int Rev Cytol 1980 (68): 251-300

73 Dive C, Evans CE, Whetton AD: Induction of apoptosis - new targets for cancer chemotherapy. Sem Cancer Biology 1992 (3):417-427

74 Raff M: Social controls on cell survival and death. Nature 1992 (356):397-400

75 Fanidi A, Harrington EA, Evan GI: Cooperative interaction between c-*myc* and *bcl*-2 oncogene. Nature 1992 (359):554-556

76 Workman P and Graham MA: Pharmacokinetics of Cancer Chemotherapy. Cancer Surveys, Vol 17. Cold Spring Harbor, 1993

77 Zachary I and Rozengurt E: Focal adhesion kinase (p125^{FAK}): A point of convergence in the action of neuropeptides, integrins and oncogenes. Cell 1992 (71):891-894

78 Weiner TM, Liu EJ, Craven RJ Cance WG: Expression of focal adhesion kinase gene and invasive cancer. Lancet 1993 (342):1024-1025

79 Millauer B, Shawver LK, Plate KH, Risan W, Ullrich A: Glioblastoma growth inhibited in vivo by a dominant-negative flk-1 mutant. Nature 1994 (367):576-579

Apoptosis and Cancer Therapy

Wilfried Bursch

Institut für Tumorbiologie-Krebsforschung der Universität Wien, Borschkegasse 8a, 1090 Vienna, Austria

Cell death is an important and widespread phenomenon in biology. It serves to shape the final form of organisms during embryonic development and metamorphosis [1-3] and it counterbalances cell generation in tissues. Disturbance of its control can lead to malformation [4-6] or carcinogenesis [7,8]. Cell death is also a significant result of tissue damage and a cause of disease [9]. Moreover, its induction is the goal of most current strategies for cancer therapy. Recently, new concepts have emerged related to the different types of cell death occurring in this wide variety of circumstances.

In 1972 J. Kerr, A. Wyllie and A. Currie proposed a classification of cell death into 2 broad categories. They introduced the term *apoptosis* to describe a type of cell death *"which appears to play a complementary but opposite role to mitosis in the regulation of animal cell populations. Its morphological features suggest that it is an active, inherently programmed phenomenon"* which can be *"initiated or inhibited by a variety of environmental stimuli, both physiological and pathological"* [10]. Necrosis, according to this proposal, is usually *"determined not by factors intrinsic to the cell itself, but by environmental perturbation, which must be violent"* leading to rapid incapacitation of major cell functions (gene expression, ATP synthesis, membrane potential) and to collapse of internal homeostasis [10,11]. Necrosis is associated with membrane lysis and inflammation [9], which may trigger potentially dangerous secondary responses within the organism. Extensive necrosis can damage the structure of a tissue. In spite of these functional implications the emphasis in the definition of apoptosis and its discrimination from necrosis were based on morphological criteria.

Apoptosis occurs through a series of morphologically distinct alterations which include shrinkage of cytoplasm, condensation of chromatin and fragmentation of the affected cell into membrane-bound "apoptotic bodies" [10] (Fig. 1,2). A basic feature of apoptosis under many circumstances is that the dying cell and its fragments are secluded by intact membranes until the final stage of digestion after phagocytosis. Thereby, and in contrast to lytic cell death (necrosis), liberation of potentially harmful substances such as DNA, antigens, and eicosanoids, activation of macrophages with formation of oxygen radicals, inflammation etc. may be avoided. Thus, from a teleological

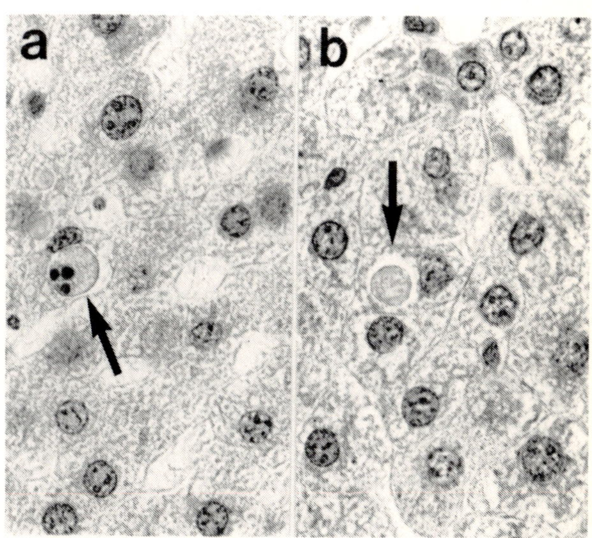

Fig. 1. Morphological signs of apoptosis in rat liver. (a) extra-hepatocellular apoptotic body with chromatin (↑); (b) intra-hepatocellular apoptotic body without chromatin (↑). (Hematoxylin-eosin, x600)

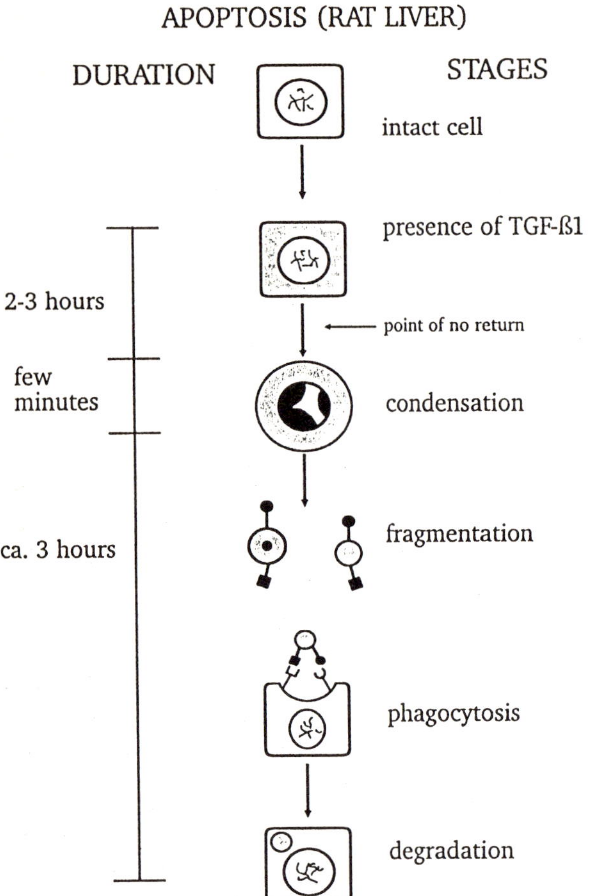

Fig. 2. Stages and duration of apoptosis in rat liver. The figure is explained in the text. Data are taken from references 61 and 116. The point of no return is defined by the appearance of resistance to mitogen-induced cell rescue [16].

point of view, apoptosis appears to be more advantageous for removal of injured cells than necrosis [10,11]. Interestingly, surface molecules such as lectin binding sites [12], vitronectin receptor [13], phosphatidylserine [14] or asialoglycoprotein receptor [15] were found to be involved in recognition and removal of apoptotic cells.

The concept of apoptosis is attracting increasing attention and has provided new insights into the control and function of cell death in a variety of (patho)physiological states [16-18]. Elucidation of factors and mechanisms involved in the regulation of apoptosis will help to better understand tumour development and, on the other hand, should also open new strategies for preventive and curative therapy of cancer.

Apoptosis: Incidence and Function in the Pathogenesis of Diseases

Apoptosis does not appear to occur at random in all cells of a tissue. Old, preneoplastic, damaged, autoreactive or excessive cells can be eliminated preferentially [16-18]. Such a selectivity in apoptosis may provide a basis for its protective role against disease. Either inappropiate induction or inhibition of apoptosis can have deleterious effects for the organism, a topic which has been extensively reviewed elsewhere [16-18]. There is a growing body of evidence showing that inhibition of apoptotic elimination of potentially harmful cells appears to be one of the key mechanisms in the pathogenesis of autoimmune diseases and neoplasia.

During maturation of the immune system, clones of autoreactive T-lymphocytes bearing high-affinity T-cell receptors for self-antigens are deleted via apoptosis [19,20]. In a transgenic mouse model, self-reactive Ly-1B cells, which express an anti-erythrocyte autoantibody, are deleted by apoptosis when exposed to the self-antigen *in vivo* [21]. However, some of these cells can escape from the apoptotic deletion mechanism. This cell population is considered to expand in the peritoneal cavity, i.e., a microenvironment lacking the self-antigen, eventually causing haemolytic anaemia [21]. These examples show that cell death by apoptosis is a very important mechanism to prevent autoimmune diseases.

Inhibition of apoptosis may also underly the teratogenic effects of certain chemicals [4-6,22]. Prenatal exposure of mice to diethylstilboestrol (DES) seems to inhibit the physiological regression of sexual anlagen [23]. The role of apoptosis in this process has not yet been elucidated; the regression of sexual anlagen possibly occurs through an autophagic, lysosomal-driven type of cell death as described by Schweichel and Merker [22]. The persistence of the duct is considered to result in malformation of the male genital tract including lesions that resemble neoplasia [24].

Apoptosis has been found to modulate the stages of initiation, promotion and progression in the stepwise formation of cancer in the liver and other organs. The biologically-based mathematical model of Moolgavkar predicts an 80-90% cell loss of initiated (preneoplastic) cells from the liver [25]. The first experimental evidence that newly formed preneoplastic cells in rat liver are efficiently eliminated was provided by A. Columbano et al. [26]. These studies indicated that regression of mitogen-induced liver hyperplasia almost completely inhibited expansion of preneoplastic foci, probably due to preferential elimination of focal cells via apoptosis. In studies by Schulte-Hermann et al. the fate of initiated liver cells as visualised by glutathione-S-transferase (GST-P) was followed closely during the first 4 weeks after a necrogenic dose of N-nitrosomorpholine [27]. A rapid upsurge of GST-P-positive single hepatocytes during regenerative hepatocellular proliferation was followed by a decline to approximately 20% of the peak value. The disappearance of single GST-P-positive cells is obviously not due to cell division resulting in focal cell populations consisting of 2 and more cells. Although it is not yet proven that the GST-P-positive cells are truly initiated and that they disappear only through apoptosis, these findings suggest that initiation as indicated by the occurrence of cells with an altered phenotype is not as stable as is usually assumed.

In the promotion stage, the rate of apoptosis was found to be a rate-limiting factor for the growth of the preneoplastic cell populations. An early observation was that putative preneoplastic foci exhibited much higher rates of cell proliferation than normal liver but showed almost no net growth during several months [7,28]. With tumour promoters (non-genotoxic carcinogens) such as α-hexachlorocyclohexane or phenobarbital (PB), foci growth could be dramatically enhanced without persistent significant enhancement of cell proliferation. Closer analysis of this phenomenon revealed that apoptosis counterbalanced the enhanced rate of cell replication. PB (and other tumour promoters) can inhibit apoptosis in liver foci and thereby accelerate their growth and the occurrence of frank neoplasia [7,28]. Furthermore, the rate of apoptoses was inversely correlated with the stability of the expression of the altered phenotype [28]. It is also noteworthy that in the absence of treatment with a tumour promoter preneoplastic foci exhibited a slow growth in later stages (after about 7 months). Conceivably, the high cell turnover in the early foci may result in selection of preneoplastic cell populations that gradually may evade the apoptotic defense mechanism. On the other hand, stimulation of apoptosis in preneoplastic foci of the liver by S-adenosyl-L-methionine resulted in prevention of heptocarcinogenesis [29].

Inhibition of apoptosis appears to be a pathogenic mechanism of general importance as it occurs not only in the liver, but also in other organs. Studies on breast biopsies of premenopausal women suggested that a decreased rate in apoptotic elimination of breast epithelial cells is associated with the occurrence of fibrocytic change and increased risk of carcinoma development [30]. Inhibition of apoptotic elimination of B-cells due to overexpression of the oncogene *bcl*-2 is involved in the pathogenesis of Burkitt lymphoma [18,31,32]. Furthermore, the adenovirus E1A can initiate the transformation of primary rodent cells which, however, subsequently die by apoptosis [33]. Survival of the transformed cells and formation of foci requires expression of additional proteins, namely E1B 19K or E1B 55K which block apoptosis. Likewise, overexpression of *bcl*-2 also was found to inhibit apoptosis under these conditions [33,34].

Apoptosis also occurs at later stages of carcinoma development such as neoplastic nodules and also quite frequently in untreated experimental and human tumours [35]. Kinetic studies on a murine sarcoma revealed that apoptosis can considerably contribute to cell loss from this tumour [36]. These observations suggest that apoptosis provides a target for therapeutic intervention which is as important as the more commonly considered biochemistry of cell proliferation.

Apoptosis: A Network of Extrinsic and Intrinsic Factors Involved in the Induction of Cell Death and a Potential Target for Therapeutic Intervention

The pioneering work of G. Beatson [37] and C. Huggins [38] showed that surgical ablation of trophic hormones can cause regression of hormone-dependent tumours. These observations paved the way for the development of the hormonal therapy of neoplasia. There is accumulating evidence showing that surgical or chemical ablation of trophic hormones not only reduces cell proliferation but also triggers apoptosis. An oestrogen-dependent kidney tumour showed rapid growth with diethylstilboestrol (DES); withdrawal of DES caused tumour regression and retreatment induced tumour growth again [39]. In the growth period a high mitotic activity and a relatively low number of apoptoses was found; the opposite occurred during tumour regression after DES withdrawal. It should be noted that large necrotic areas were also present in these tumours. The incidence of these necrotic areas did not, however, change in the presence or absence of DES. Thus the actual growth rate of the tumour predominantly depended on the ratio between proliferation and apoptosis [39]. The LH-RH analogue D-Trp-6-LH-RH, the LH-RH antagonist SB-75 and the somatostatin analogue RC-160 led to massive apoptosis and regression of chemically induced pancreatic cancer in hamsters; combination of these compounds or of either compound with 5-fluorouracil has been found to increase the efficiency of the therapy of pancreatic tumours [40,41]. The LH-RH antagonist SB-75 was also shown to cause regression of human prostate carcinoma (PC-82) xenografts in nude mice by inhibition of cell proliferation and induction of apoptosis [42]. Furthermore, progesterone antagonists exerted a tumour-inhibiting effect in various hormone-dependent mammary tumour models; the antitumour activity of antiprogestins is considered to result from induction of terminal differentiation leading to apoptosis of the tumour cells [43]. *In vivo* studies with the human prostate PC-82 and the mammary cancer cell line MCF-7 revealed that ablation of androgen and oestrogen, respectively, induced apoptosis and tumour regression [44,45]. Likewise, in MCF-7 cell cultures tamoxifen and other anti-oestrogens induced both a depression of DNA synthesis and an increase in cell death [Kienzl and Bursch, unpubl.]. To what extent induction of cell death may contribute to the preventive effect of tamoxifen against mammary cancer development in patients at risk remains to be elucidated. Conceivably, this could result from anti-promotion by the antagonist via induction of apoptosis in cancer prestages. Apoptosis may also have general importance in therapy of human lymphatic leukaemia as suggested by glucocorticoid-induced apoptosis of normal and transformed haematological cells [11,17-20] as

well as by the induction of death of these cells through cytostatic drugs (see below).

A major aggravation for hormonal tumour therapy of endocrine organs and leukaemia results from the selection of hormone-independent and glucocorticoid-resistant cells. In various haematological cell lines apoptosis cannot be induced by glucocorticoids because of reduced receptor affinity or due to a lack of receptors [46]. Likewise, selection of mammary tumour cells with down-regulated oestrogen-receptor expression appears to limit the efficiency of adjuvant tamoxifen therapy [47]. On the other hand, the conversion from oestrogen-dependent to independent tumour cells may include mutations of the steroid-receptor leading to its permanent activation [48]. Transcriptional control may be knocked out as a result of this. Interestingly, retinoic acid-induced apoptosis of human squamous carcinoma cells was found to involve signal transduction via the steroid receptor-like α-type retinoic acid receptor [49]. Recently, oncogenes (c-*myc* and others, see below) were found to be involved in the initiation of apoptosis. These findings may provide new experimental approaches to elucidate how tumour cells escape from apoptosis control.

Apoptosis has also been found to be mediated by receptors belonging to the nerve growth factor/tumour necrosis factor (NGF/TNF) superfamily. Tumor necrosis factor-α (TNF-α) was found to induce apoptosis in mammary adenocarcinoma cell lines [50], a human monocyte-like cell line U937 [51] and primary rat hepatocyte cultures [52]. However, TNF-α also appears to be able to stimulate different pathways of cell death. Depending on the target cell, TNF-α may induce an incomplete apoptotic programme or may even lead to necrosis [53]. Other studies showed that antibodies directed against cell surface molecules, namely anti-Fas [54] and anti-Apo1 [55], were capable of inducing apoptosis in malignant human lymphatic cell lines as well as fresh human leukaemic cells. Recently, sequence analysis revealed that the Fas and Apo-1 antigen are identical and that this molecule exhibits a significant similarity to the NGF/TNF receptor superfamily [56]. Fas/Apo-1 may open new ways for a selective use of antibodies in therapy because its expression in Burkitt lymphoma cell lines was found to correlate with a shift towards the lymphoblastoid phenotype [57]. The mRNA transcribing the Fas antigen was also found to be expressed in mouse thymus, liver and heart, but not in brain and spleen [58]. Therefore, future studies might reveal that the Fas/Apo1 antigen provides a target for the induction of apoptosis in other cell types. Furthermore, new techniques for antibody production such as the phage system (see R. Hawkins, this volume) will certainly stimulate efforts to refine antibody therapy.

Recently, transforming growth factor-ß1 (TGF-ß1) was recognised as a physiological factor which plays an important role within the regulatory network that controls the balance between replication and death in the endometrium and the liver [59-61]. *In vivo* studies showed that apoptotic hepatocytes in normal and preneoplastic liver exhibited immunostaining for TGF-ß1. The staining was much stronger with antibodies recognising the latency-associated protein (LAP; dimer of the pro-region non-covalently associated with the mature region) rather than the mature peptide itself [61]. This may be explained by the biological half-life of the pre-form of TGF ß1, which is about 2 hours, whereas that of the mature TGF-ß1 is only 2 minutes. Thus, once mature TGF-ß1 is released from the precursor by proteolytic cleavage, its rapid degradation may result in low levels in the cells that may be insufficient for detection under the experimental conditions used [61]. However, the presence of TGF-ß1 in apoptotic cells alone did not prove that it is truly involved in the regulation of this type of cell death. Further studies with primary hepatocyte cultures as well as *in vivo* studies with regressing rat liver revealed that TGF-ß1 does indeed induce apoptosis [60,61]. In these studies, however, the mature form of TGF-ß1 was much more potent in the induction of apoptosis than its precursor [60]. Taken together the *in vitro* and *in vivo* results, induction of apoptosis may be brought about either through the uptake of the precursor form by the mannose-6-phosphate/insulin-like growth factor II receptor, which is expressed in hepatocytes *in vivo* and *in vitro* [62,63] or, alternatively, TGF-ß1 may be produced by hepatocytes in its pre-form and, upon cleavage of the mature molecule, apoptosis is induced in these cells. To date, the significance of TGF-ß1 for tumour therapy is not yet clear. TGF-ß1 was found to induce apoptosis in cultured human hepatoma and gastric carcinoma cells [64,65]. Some tumour cells were found to produce TGF-ß1 but to be resistant to its growth inhibitory effects [66]. Breast tumours of patients growing despite tamoxifen treatment showed high levels of TGF-ß1 mRNA levels and clinically insignificant amounts of oestrogen receptors [67]. Likewise, TGF-ß1 also did not affect the growth of the oestrogen-receptor-negative human breast cancer line MDA-MB-231 *in vivo* [68]. Hypothetically, tumours may escape from growth restriction active on normal tissues and at the same time could prevent growth or even induce death of their healthy neighbour cells.

Recent studies on oncogene expression have revealed exciting insights into the genetic control of apoptosis and will almost certainly lead to the discovery of new targets for chemotherapy. Early growth response genes have been found to be involved in the regulation of both cell proliferation and apoptosis. In cell culture studies with rat-1 fibroblasts it was shown that c-*myc* expression is a *sufficient* condition for stimulation of cell proliferation [69]. Furthermore, c-*myc* expression was found to be a *necessary* condition for the induction of rat-1 fibroblast apoptosis. However, apoptosis also requires additional factors which are provided by serum deprivation [69]. Expression of c-*myc* is also necessary but not sufficient for the induction of apoptosis of immature T cells and T cell hybridomas after activation of the T-cell receptor complex because an antisense oligonucleotide complementary to c-*myc* was found to prevent apoptosis [70]. On the other hand, this antisense oligonucleotide failed to prevent dexamethasone-induced apoptosis of the same cells. This result is consistent with the concept that the glucocorticoid and T-cell receptors stimulate different pathways leading to apoptosis [71]. Evidence for the involvement of c-*myc* in the regulation of apoptosis has also been provided by *in vivo* studies. During the regression of rat prostate after castration, c-*myc* was found to be expressed coordinately with c-*fos* and *hsp*-70 [72,73]. However, it is not yet clear whether c-*fos* and *hsp*-70 are specifically involved in the regulation of apoptosis. Thus, in the studies with immature T cells and T-cell hybridomas, T-cell receptor mediated apoptosis could not be blocked by an antisense oligonucleotide against c-*fos* [71]. On the other hand, recent studies with a *fos-LacZ* transgenic mouse provided evidence that constitutive *fos* expression occurs in mineralising cartilage cells that are destined to die [74].

Once a given cell is stimulated by c-*myc* expression to enter the cell cycle, additional signals at certain stages direct the cell either to undergo apoptosis or to complete the cycle. At the transcriptional level, *in vivo* and *in vitro* studies with haematopoietic cells revealed that the proto-oncogene *bcl*-2, which encodes a protein of the inner mitochondrial membrane, is a negative regulator of apoptosis. *Bcl*-2 is differentially expressed during T cell maturation and blocks the apoptotic elimination of immature thymocytes [17,18,75]. Thus, in the thymus *bcl*-2 expression is confined to mature thymocytes of the medulla; likewise, in the germinal centres it is confined to zones of surviving B cells [75]. Studies with certain B-cell lineages (FDC-P1, LyH7) suggest that *bcl*-2 cooperates with c-*myc*, i.e., *bcl*-2 acts as a survival signal and c-*myc* serves for expansion of the respective B cell population [31]. Chromosomal translocation results in overexpression of *bcl*-2 and block of apoptosis in certain B and T cell lines in a cell type and/or factor-restricted fashion [18]. Likewise, c-*myc* and *bcl*-2 cooperate in apoptosis of Chinese hamster ovary cells [76]. Deregulation of *bcl*-2 expression may allow a cell to survive growth factor deprivation and expand selectively; thereby, the probability of acquiring further genetic changes and the subsequent development of frank neoplasia will be increased. Overexpression of *bcl*-2 may also limit chemotherapy as *bcl*-2 protects CD4+8+ thymocytes from glucocorticoid, radiation and CD3 induced apoptosis [77]. Likewise, EBV-transformed cells became resistant to tentandrine, a bisbenzylisoquinoline alkaloid with anti-inflammatory activity [78]. It is worth noting that the function of the mammalian *bcl*-2 gene as a negative regulator of apoptosis corresponds to that of the *ced*-9 gene known to regulate programmed cell death in the nematode *C. elegans* [79]. Future studies will probably reveal a structural homology between these genes.

Another gene found to be involved in the control of apoptosis is the tumour suppressor gene *p53*. The wild type form of this gene was found to induce apoptosis of myeloid leukaemic cells, while mutation resulting in loss of *p53* activity causes resistance to the induction of apoptosis [80]. Deregulation of *p53* may also be involved in human hepatocarcinogenesis as 50% of the cases of primary hepatocellular carcinoma in southern Africa exhibit a mutation of this gene [81]. Furthermore, blood analysis of patients suffering from acute myeloid leukaemia suggests that changes in *p53* protein conformation without point mutation may also cause its malfunction [82]. It is assumed that the wild-type *p53* protein blocks cells in G_1, either allowing the cell to repair damaged DNA or to direct it into apoptosis; thereby, transmission of damaged DNA to progeny cells is prevented [83-86]. In the context of this review, it should be noted that in a recent study with a human colon tumour cell line (EB), stimulation of wild-type *p53* expression results in apoptosis and tumour regression [87].

It should be emphasised that a number of other genes were found to be involved in the induction and completion of cell death. This has been reviewed recently by Ellis, Yuan and Horvitz [79] and will not be discussed further here.

In summary, there is substantial evidence that at the transcriptional level regulation of cell proliferation and apoptosis are closely associated (Fig. 3). Expression of c-*myc* may stimulate the cell to enter the cell cycle and thereby prime it for apoptosis. *Bcl*-2 may provide a survival factor while *p53* may provide a death factor. In concert, these genes determine whether a given cell either undergoes apoptosis or completes the cycle. At the epigenetic level, survival signals may be provided by the serum as exemplified by the studies on rat-1 fibroblast apoptosis [70]. In haematological cells, interleukins have been shown to act as survival factors [17-20]. This concept is in full agreement with early observations suggesting that inhibition of apoptosis by cell or tissue-specific mitogens such as ACTH, nerve growth factor, erythropoietin and liver tumour promoter is a fundamental characteristic of this type of cell death; it may even be used to discriminate apoptosis from other forms of cell death [11,16]. The recent concepts of genetic control of apoptosis provide a challenge for the development of antisense and antigene drugs [88, S. Neidle, this volume]. Thus, in a human squamous cell carcinoma cell line (SCC-25), antisense DNA complementary for the α-type retinoic acid receptor mRNA is considered to induce apoptosis [49].

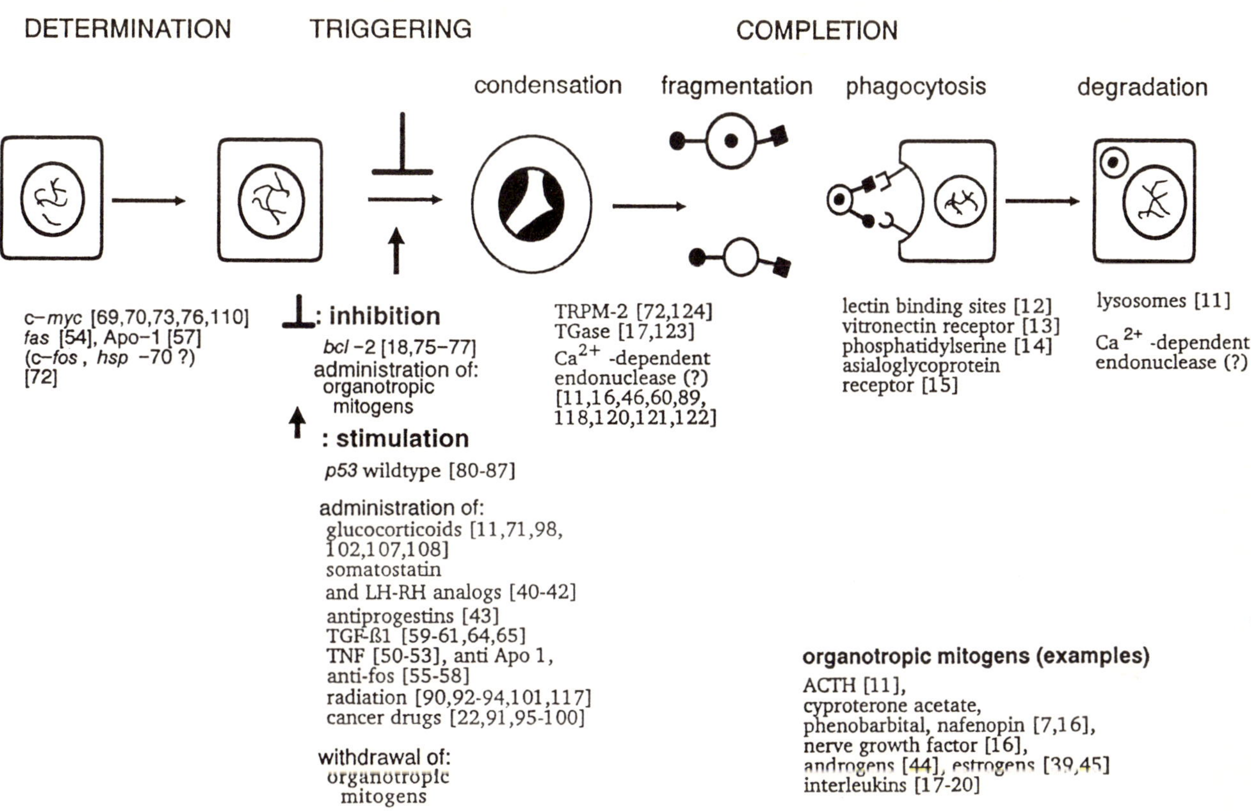

Fig. 3. Genes and factors involved in the induction and completion of apoptosis. The figure is explained in the text. In brackets: references

Cytostatic Drugs and Irradiation

Cytostatic drugs and irradiation may also activate apoptosis. Morphological evidence of apoptosis has been obtained in the liver, intestine and bone marrow after exposure to cytarabine, nitrogen mustard, diethylnitrosamine (DENA) and other compounds as well as after irradiation [22,89-91]. In lymphatic cells, DNA fragmentation readily occurs after radiation or various cancer drugs such as cisplatin, etoposide, aphidicolin, camptothecin, hydroxyurea and other compounds [92-100]. However, it is not yet clear whether this reflects the activation of the complete apoptotic programme or if so, how apoptosis is initiated in the affected cell.

There is little information on how DNA damage could trigger the programme of events eventually resulting in apoptosis. A recognition process may be involved and further signal transduction may include an increase in cytosolic Ca^{2+} levels and inositol trisphosphate synthesis [96]. Studies with human B-cell (BM 13674) and T-cell (CEM-C7) lymphoid tumour cell lines suggested that radiation-induced apoptosis is associated with activation of phosphorylase 1, 2A and to a lesser extent 2B, resulting in a specific dephosphorylation pattern [101]. Protein kinase C (PKC) seems also to participate in signal transduction leading to cell death. Activation of PKC can prevent apoptosis of thymocytes induced by glucocorticoid [102] or of GM-SF and IL-3-dependent haemopoietic cells after growth factor deprivation [103]. On the other hand, activation of PKC may also participate in a pathway leading to apoptosis, as suggested by studies on TCR/CD3 complex-induced apoptosis of T-cell hybridomas [71]. Correspondingly, inhibition of PKC was also found to inhibit irradiation-induced apoptosis of murine thymocytes [104]. These findings clearly indicate that PKC is involved in the signal transduction pathway leading to cell death and is a potential target for modulating the responsiveness of cells for the induction of apoptosis [105]; however, its role does not appear to be unique in different biological conditions. These observations should stimulate a closer study of the role of PKC and other enzymes involved in signal transduction pathways leading to apoptosis, e.g. those involving tyrosine kinases (see P. Workman; G. Powis, this volume).

In lymphocytes, an intimate relationship seems to exist between DNA damage, DNA repair capacity and cell viability. It has been suggested that cessation of DNA repair as indicated by arrest of poly(ADP-ribose-) synthesis causes accumulation of DNA damage that eventually might activate apoptosis [106]. Likewise, inhibition of poly(ADP-ribose-) synthesis was found to increase the rate of apoptosis in glucocorticoid-treated S.49 lymphoma cells [107]. Recent results provided further evidence that poly-(ADP-ribosyl)ation and DNA fragmentation in lymphocytes are closely associated [108,109]. The topoisomerase-II-inhibitor teniposide was found to induce DNA strand breaks in the human HL-60 leukaemia and HT-29 colon carcinoma cell lines [110]. The primary DNA damage was followed by secondary DNA fragmentation into oligonucleosomes indicative of apoptosis in the HL-60, but this did not occur in the HT-29 cell line. This result is consistent with the requirement of c-*myc* for the initiation of apoptosis in some cell types (see above) since HL-60 exhibits an amplified c-*myc* expression but HT-29 does not [110].

The extent of DNA/cell damage appears to determine whether apoptosis or necrosis will occur. In rat liver high doses of DENA seemed to cause predominantly necrosis, whereas low doses predominantly induced apoptosis [111]. After CCl_4 exposure pericentral hepatocytes undergo lytic cell death (necrosis), whereas at least some of the periportal hepatocytes enter apoptosis, as indicated by morphological features and a positive immunostaining for TGF-ß1 [61]. Conceivably, periportal cells generate less toxic metabolites from CCl_4 than pericentral hepatocytes, and these are insufficient for immediate breakdown of internal homeostasis but can stimulate apoptosis [112]. Likewise, in a study with murine mastocytoma cells, moderate hyperthermia induced apoptosis, while

more intense hyperthermia caused necrosis [113]. Thus a critical dose of injury may exist beyond which necrosis occurs in a given cell. Whether or not a cell enters apoptosis may also depend on factors related to the cell cycle. Early observations in mouse intestine after radiation or cancer drugs (e.g. 5-fluorouracil, vincristine, actinomycin D) showed that crypt cells of the proliferating cell pool preferentially underwent apoptosis, whereas most cells from the non-proliferating pool survived [90]. Furthermore, Chinese hamster V79 fibroblasts enter apoptosis after cold shock treatment at the transition between the logarithmic and stationary growth phase. Likewise, Chinese hamster ovary cells underwent apoptosis in response to cancer drugs such as cisplatin after G_2-M arrest [114]. Recent studies with T-cell hybridomas treated with cancer drugs such as actinomycin, camptothecin or aphidicolin suggested that apoptosis can be induced in all phases of the cell cycle; in the case of the topoisomerase 1 inhibitor camptothecin, cells in G_1 were most sensitive [97]. On the other hand, camptothecin was found to induce apoptosis of HL-60 cells selectively in the S-phase [115]. Furthermore, rat thymocytes were found to enter apoptosis after glucocorticoids or camptothecin only in G_0, whereas proliferating cells were resistant [98]. Irradiation of murine T-cell hybridoma appears to result in oxidative DNA damage and the affected cells enter apoptosis in the G_1 phase of the cell cycle subsequent to irradiation [94]; it may well be that this sequence of DNA damage and occurrence of apoptosis involves *p53* activity. Taken together, these observations show that cell cycle-specific factors can modify the initiation of apoptosis. However, there appears to be no universal response pattern to chemotherapeutic agents among the different phenotypes of tumour cells.

In conclusion, heterogeneous pathways leading to DNA fragmentation and apoptosis obviously exist, but are poorly understood at present. Studies comparing various toxins, cell types, *in vivo* and cell culture conditions, dose-dependency and kinetics of cell death etc. are needed to help elucidate the underlying mechanisms.

Detection of Apoptosis and its Discrimination from Other Types of Cell Death

The classification of a subtype of cell death as apoptosis may contain inherent difficulties because of the paucity of markers suited for proper discrimination. The morphological features of apoptosis (Fig. 1,2) have been widely used, predominantly in the field of pathology. The typical condensation of chromatin at the nuclear membrane can be detected at the electron- and light-microscopical level and may well be used as an indicator of apoptosis. *In vitro*, chromatin condensation was found to be a reliable marker for quantitative detection of apoptosis as it lasts about 90 minutes in primary hepatocyte cultures [60]. *In vivo*, however, this stage of apoptosis may last only a few minutes. Its occurrence is rare *in vivo* [116] and therefore of limited use for quantitative analysis. Apoptotic cell residues (apoptotic bodies) are more frequently encountered in tissues. At the electron-microscopical level the distinction of apoptotic bodies from other types of cell death may be unequivocal. This is not always the case at the light-microscopical level and requires great experience. Furthermore, in rat liver apoptotic bodies once formed are eliminated within less than 3 hours [116] (Fig. 2). A similar duration was found in mouse intestine, where occurrence and disappearance of apoptotic bodies was studied after irradation [117]. On the other hand, in the adrenal cortex a duration of apoptosis of 18 hours was noted [11]. Thus, in certain tissues only a low number of morphological signs of apoptosis at any given time point may be found, in spite of a high rate of cell elimination.

An early metabolic change associated with apopotosis is considered to be the activation of a non-lysosomal endonuclease, which cuts chromatin into oligonucleosomes [118]. The resulting chromatin fragmentation yields a characteristic ladder pattern after gel electrophoresis and is frequently used to detect apoptosis, so far mostly in thymocytes and lymphocytes. However, endonuclease activation may not always be obligatory for apoptosis [119,120]. Furthermore, morphologically proven apoptosis in hepatocytes and other epithelial cells can occur without DNA fragmentation into oligonucleosomes [60]. The absence of detectable DNA fragmentation in *individual* apoptotic nuclei was further verified by *in situ* nick translation, not only in hepatocytes but also in a mouse lymphoma cell line [120]. Furthermore, endonuclease is constitutively present in intact, non-apoptotic nuclei and may also be activated by mechanisms *not* related to apoptosis but to necrosis [121] or post-mortem in lytic cells [122]. Thus, the general occurrence of DNA fragmentation into oligonucleosomes during apoptosis in different cell types has not been established. Therefore, endonuclease activation should not be considered as a *general* marker of apoptosis.

Further biochemical markers for apoptosis may be the expression of transglutaminase, which cross-links glutamine and lysine residues in proteins and may serve to seal the membrane of apoptotic cells/fragments [123]. Another promising marker is the testosterone-repressed prostate message (TRPM-2) which is expressed in various tissues (e.g. prostate, liver) during involution; the product is probably sulphated glycoprotein-2 (SGP-2) [124].

Recent findings suggest that TGF-ß1 precursor seems to be present in apoptotic but not in necrotic hepatocytes, and so immunostaining for this protein may become a useful marker of apoptosis and even of pre-apoptotic cells [61] (Fig. 2).

The discrimination between apoptosis and necrosis may also be rendered difficult by incomplete expression of the genes involved in apoptosis. This may result in a necrotic appearance of dead cells. Because cell culture systems are widely used to study apoptosis, the possible occurrence of transitions between both processes is of practical importance: a cell may begin on a pathway to apoptotic death but then collapse completely and terminate in necrosis ("secondary necrosis"); this readily occurs in cell cultures where apoptotic cells are not phagocytosed as they are in tissues.

Furthermore, the dichotomy of the morphological features of apoptosis and necrosis does not appear to be applicable to all biological conditions. It is worth noting that in 1973 Schweichel and Merker [22] described morphological features of cell death denoted "type 1" which meet exactly with those denoted as apoptosis by Kerr et al. [reviewed by Clarke, 125]. In addition, Schweichel and Merker described an autophagic type of cell death ("type 2"). It does not start with condensation of the nucleus but is driven by the lysosomes of the dying cell. The lysosomal-driven cell death is completed, like the type 1 cell death, by phagocytosis of cell fragments by neighbouring cells. Type 2 cell death occurs, for example, during embryogenesis when large tissue areas or organ anlagen are removed *in toto* (e.g. cavity formation in intestine, regression of sexual anlagen). Interestingly, recent electron-microscopical studies on tamoxifen-induced cell death in MCF-7 breast tumour cell cultures also suggest the involvement of lysosomes in early stages of cell death [Kienzl, Ellinger and Bursch, unpubl.]. Furthermore, oestrogen was found to inhibit tamoxifen-induced death of MCF-7 cells and this functional criterion is suggestive of apoptosis [16]. Closer studies of this phenomenon might reveal that apoptosis/type 1 and the lysosomal-driven type 2 cell death share some regulatory steps before its morphological manifestation.

Originally, apoptosis was defined on the basis of morphological and functional grounds. Unfortunately, at present no biochemical or molecular alteration is known that could serve as a general marker of apoptosis in all different cell types. As a result, the various morphological criteria, i.e., condensation of chromatin at the nuclear membrane (detected by electron and light microscopy) and the presence of intact organelles in dead cells or cell fragments remain the best methods for identification and quantification of cell death by apoptosis. Functional (e.g. inhibition by cell/tissue-specific mitogens) and biochemical characteristics may serve as supportive evidence.

Concluding Remarks

The findings on cell death reviewed herein show that a number of heterogeneous pathways can lead to the manifestation of morphologically detectable stages of apoptosis. Furthermore, the recent developments on the network of extrinsic and intrinsic factors controlling apoptosis are revealing numerous potential targets for therapeutic intervention. Receptor and signal transduction pathways may be used for selective induction of apoptosis in target cells. Thus a number of synthetic hormone agonists and antagonists as well as some antibodies have already been shown to induce apoptosis. Furthermore, therapeutic modulation of the signal transduction pathways in tumour cells might facilitate the induction of apoptosis by hormones, antibodies and, moreover, cytostatic drugs. The genetic control of apoptosis should attract researchers in the field of antisense/antigene drug development. A growing body of evidence suggests that expression of c-*myc* may prime some normal and transformed cells for apoptosis. This gene exhibits deregulated expressions in a considerable number of tumour cell types. Moreover, the decision as to whether such cells enter the apoptosis versus the proliferation pathway appears to be dependent on the control by additional signals such as those provided by the *bcl*-2 and *p53* genes. Therefore, these genes and their products seem to be particulary promising targets for antigene/antisense drugs to block proliferation and to direct cells into apoptosis. Low-molecular-weight chemical drugs capable of this function may also be envisaged. As outlined above, many or even most of the features of apoptosis are not yet understood at the molecular level. However, our present knowledge clearly shows that apoptosis is an important endpoint in testing new cancer drugs and the outcome of future studies in this exciting area of research may help to improve the efficiency of chemotherapy.

REFERENCES

1   Glücksmann A: Cell death in normal vertebrate ontogeny. Biol Rev Cambridge Phil Soc 1951 (26):59-86

2   Lockshin RA and Williams CM: Programmed cell death. II. Endocrine potentiation of the breakdown of the intersegmental muscles of silkmoths. J Insect Physiol 1964 (10):643-649

3   Saunders JW: Death in embryonic systems death of cells is the usual accompaniment of embryonic growth and differentiation. Science 1966 (154):604-612

4   Goldman AS, Baker MK, Piddington R and Herold R: Inhibition of programmed cell death in mouse embryonic palate *in vitro* by cortisol and phenytoin: receptor involvement and requirement of protein synthesis. Proc Soc Exp Biol Med 1983 (174):239-243

5   Sulik KK and Dehart DB: Retinoic acid-induced limb malformations resulting from apical ectodermal ridge cell death. Teratology 1988 (37):527-537

6   Manson JM and Miller ML: Contribution of mesenchymal cell death and mitotic alteration to asymmetric limb malformations induced by MNNG. Teratogenesis Carcinogenesis and Mutagenesis 1983 (3):335-353

7   Bursch W, Lauer B, Timmermann-Trosiener I, Barthel G, Schuppler J and Schulte-Hermann R: Controlled cell death (apoptosis) of normal and putative preneoplastic cells in rat liver following withdrawal of tumor promoters. Carcinogenesis 1984 (5):453-458

8   Columbano A, Ledda-Columbano GM, Rao PM, Rajalakshmi S and Sarma DSR: Occurrence of cell death (apoptosis) in preneoplastic and neoplastic liver cells. Am J Pathol 1984 (116):441-446

9   Popper H and Keppler D: Networks of interacting mechanisms of hepatocellular degeneration and death. In: H Popper and F Schaffner (eds) Progress in Liver Disease, Vol. VIII. Grune and Stratton Inc, Orlando 1986 pp 209-236

10 Kerr JFR, Wyllie AH and Currie AR: Apoptosis: a basic biological phenomenon with wide-ranging implications in tissue kinetics. Br J Cancer 1972 (26):239-257

11 Wyllie AH, Kerr J and Currie A: Cell death: the significance of apoptosis. Int Rev Cytol 1980 (68):251-306

12 Wyllie AH, Morris RG, Smith AL and Dunlop D: Hormone-induced cell death. 2. Surface changes in thymocytes undergoing apoptosis. Am J Pathol 1984 (115):426-436

13 Savill J, Dransfield I, Hogg N and Haslett Ch: Vitronectin receptor-mediated phagocytosis of cells undergoing apoptosis. Nature 1990 (343):170-173

14 Fadok VA, Voelker DR, Campbell PA, Cohen JJ, Bratton DL and Henson PM: Exposure of phosphatidlyserine on the surface of apoptotic bodies triggers specific recognition and removal by macrophages. J Immunol 1992 (148):2207-2207

15 Dini L, Autuori F, Lentini A, Oliverio S and Piancentini M: The clearance of apoptotic cells against the liver is mediated by the asialoglycoprotein receptor. FEBS Lett 1992 (296):174-178

16 Bursch W, Oberhammer F and Schulte-Hermann R: Cell death and its protective role in disease. Trends Pharm Sci 1992 (13):245-251

17 Fesus L: Apoptosis fashions T and B cell repertoire. Immunology Letters 1991 (30):277-282

18 Korsmeyer SJ: Chromosomal translocation in lymphoid malignancies reveal novel proto-oncogenes. Ann Rev Immunology 1992 (10):785-807

19 MacDonald HR and Lees RK: Programmed cell death of autoreactive thymocytes. Nature 1990 (343):642-644

20 Cohen JJ, Duke R, Fadok V and Sellins K: Apoptosis and programmed cell death in immunity. Annu Rev Immunol 1992 (10):267-293

21 Murakami M, Tsubata T, Okamoto M, Shimizu A, Kumagai S, Imura H and Honjo T: Antigen-induced apoptotic death of Ly-1B cells responsible for autoimmune disease in transgenic mice. Nature 1992 (357):77-80

22 Schweichel JU and Merker HJ: The morphology of various types of cell death in prenatal tissues. Teratology 1973 (7):253-266

23 Bullock BC, Newbold RR and McLachlan JA: Lesions associated with prenatal diethystilbestrol exposure. Env Health Persp 1988 (77).29-31

24 Newbold RR, Bullock BC and McLachlan IA: Mullerian remnants of male mice exposed prenatally to diethylstilbestrol. Teratogenesis Carcinog Mutagen 1987 (7):377-389

25 Mollgavkar SH: Multistages models for cancer risk assessment .In: Travis CC (ed) Biologically Based Models for Cancer Risk Assessment, Vol 159. Plenum Press, New York 1989 pp 9-20

26 Columbano A, Ledda-Columbano GM, Ennas MG, Curto M, Chelo A and Pani P: Cell proliferation and promotion of rat liver carcinogenesis: different effect of hepatic regeneration and mitogen induced hyperplasia on the development of enzyme-altered foci. Carcinogenesis 1990 (11):771-776

27 Schulte-Hermann R, Bursch W, Grasl-Kraupp B, Oberhammer F and Wagner A: Programmed cell death and its protective role with particular reference to apoptosis. Toxicology Letters 1992 (64/65):569-574

28 Schulte-Hermann R, Timmermann-Trosiener I, Barthel G and Bursch W: DNA synthesis, apoptosis and phenotypic expression as determinants of growth of altered foci in rat liver during phenobarbital promotion. Cancer Res 1990 (50):5127-5135

29 Pascale RM, Marras V, Simile MM, Daino L, Inna G, Bennati S, Carta M, Seddaiu MA, Massarelli G and Feo F: Chemoprevention of rat liver carcinogenesis by S- adenosyl-L-methionine: a long-term study. Cancer Res 1992 (52):4979-4986

30 Allan DJ, Howell A, Roberts SA, Wiiliams GT, Watson RJ, Coyne JD, Clarke RB, Laidlaw IJ and Potten CS: Reduction of apoptosis relative to mitosis in histologically normal epithelium accompanies fibrocystic change and carcinoma of

the premenopausal human breast. J Pathol 1992 (167):25-32

31 Vaux DL, Cory S and Adams JM: *Bcl-2* gene promotes haemopoietic cell survival and cooperates with *c-myc* to immortalize pre-B cells. Nature 1988 (335):440-442

32 Fanidi A, Harrington EA and Evan GI: Cooperative interaction between *c-myc* and *bcl-2* proto-oncogenes. Nature 1992 (359):554-556

33 White E, Sabbatini P, Debbas M, Wold WS, Kusher DI and Gooding LR: The 19-kilodalton adenovirus E1B transforming protein inhibits programmed cell death and prevents cytolysis by tumor necrosis factor alpha. Mol Cell Biol 1992 (12):2570-2580

34 Rao L, Debbas M, Sabbatini P, Hockenberry D, Korsmeyer S and White E: The adenovirus E1A proteins induce apoptosis, which is inhibited by the E1 19kDa and *bcl-2* proteins. PNAS 1992 (89):7742-7746

35 Wyllie AH: The biology of cell death in tumours. Anticancer Res 1985 (5):131-136

36 Sarraf CE and Bowen ID: Kinetic studies on a murine sarcoma and an analysis of apoptosis. Br J Cancer 1986 (54):989-998

37 Beatson GT: On the treatment of inoperable cases of carcinoma of the mamma: suggestion for a new method of treatment, with illustrative cases. Lancet 1896 (ii): 104-107

38 Huggins C, Stevens RE and Hodges CV: Studies on prostatic cancer II. The effects of castration on advanced carcinoma in the prostate gland. Arch Surg 1941 (43): 209-233

39 Bursch W, Liehr JG, Sirbasku D, Putz B, Taper H and Schulte-Hermann R: Control of cell death (apoptosis) by diethylstilbestrol in an estrogen dependent kidney tumor. Carcinogenesis 1991 (12):855-860

40 Szende B, Srkalovic G, Groot K, Lapis K and Schally AV: Regression of nitrosamine-induced pancreatic cancers in hamsters treated with luteinizing hormone-releasing hormone antagonists or agonists. Cancer Res 1990 (50):3716-3721

41 Szepeshazi K, Lapis K, Schally AV: Effect of combination treatment with analogs of luteinizing hormone-realising hormone (LH-RH) or somato-statin and 5-fluorouracil on pancreatic cancer in hamsters. Int J Cancer 1991 (49):260-26

42 Redding TW, Schally AV, Radulovic S, Milovanovic S, Szepeshazi K and Isaacs JT: Sustained release formulations of luteinizing hormone-releasing hormone antagonist SB-75 inhibit proliferation and enhance apoptotic cell death of human prostate carcinoma (PC-82) in male nude mice. Cancer Res 1992 (52):2538-2544

43 Michna H, Nishino Y, Neef G, McGuire WL and Schneider MR: Progesterone antagonists: tumor-inhibiting potential and mechanism of action. J Steroid Biochem Mol Biol 1992 (41):339-348

44 Kyprianou N, English HF and Isaacs JT: Programmed cell death during regression of PC-82 human prostate cancer following androgen abla-tion. Cancer Res 1990 (50): 3748-3753

45 Kyprianou N, English HF, Davidson NE and Isaacs JT: Programmed cell death during regression of the MCF-7 human breast cancer following estrogen ablation. Cancer Res 1991 (51):162-166

46 Wyllie AH, Morris RG, Smith AL and Dunlop D: Chromatin cleavage in apoptosis: association with condensed chromatin morphology and dependence on macromolecular synthesis. J Pathol 1984 (142):67-77

47 Early Breast Cancer Trialists' Collaborative Group: Systematic treatment of early breast cancer by hormonal, cytotoxic, or immune therapy. Lancet 1991 (339):1-15, 71-85

48 Evans RM: The steroid and thyroid hormone receptor superfamily. Science 1988 (240):889-895

49 Cope FO, Wille JJ and Tomei LD: Retinoids and retinoid receptors in malignant disease: clinical significance of their expression and the alteration of disease course with antisense DNA. Prospects for Antisense Nucleic Acid Therapy of Cancer and AIDS. Wiley-Liss Inc 1991 pp 125-141

50 Bellomo G, Perotti M, Taddei F, Mirabelli F, Finardi G, Nicotera P and Orrenius S: Tumor necrosis factor alpha induces apoptosis in mammary adenocarcinoma cells by an increase in intracel-lular free Ca^{2+} concentration and DNA fragmenta-tion. Cancer Res 1992 (52):1342-1346

51 Wright SC, Kumar P, Tam AW, Shen N, Varma M and Larrick JW: Apoptosis and DNA fragmentation precede TNF-induced cytolysis in U937 cells. J Cell Biochem 1992 (48):344-355

52 Shinagawa T, Yoshioka K, Kamuku S, Wakita T, Ishikawa T, Itoh Y and Takayanagi M: Apoptosis in cultured rat hepatocytes: the effects of tumor necrosis factor alpha and interferron gamma. J Pathol 1991 (165):247-253

53 Laster SM, Wood JG and Gooding LR: Tumor necrosis factor can induce both apoptotic and necrotic forms of cell lysis, J Immunol 1988 (141):2629-2633

54 Itoh N, Yonehara S, Ishii A, Yonehara M, Mizushima SI, Sameshima M, Hase A, Seto Y and Nagata S: The popypeptide encoded by the cDNA for human cell surface antigen fas can mediate apoptosis. Cell 1991 (66):233-234

55 Trauth BC, Klas Ch, Peters AMJ, Matzku S, Müller P, Falk W, Debatin KM and Krammer PH: Monoclonal antibody-mediated tumor regression by induction of apoptosis. Science 1989 (245):301-305

56 Oehm A, Behrmann I, Falk W, Pawlita M, Maier G, Klast C, Li-Weber M, Richards S, Dhein J, Trauth BC, Ponstingl H and Krammer PH: Purification and molecular cloning of the APO-1 cell surface antigen, a member of the tumor necrosis factor/nerve growth factor receptor superfamily. J Biol Chem 1992 (267):10709-10715

57 Falk MH, Trauth BC, Debatin KM, Klas C, Gregory CD, Rickinson AB, Calendar A, Lenoir GM, Ellwart JW and Krammer PH: Expression of the APO-1 antigen in Burkitt lymphoma cell lines correlates with a shift towards lymphoblastoid phenotype. Blood 1992 (79):3300-3306

58 Watanabe-Fukanaga R, Brannan CI, Itoh N, Yonehara S, Copeland NG, Jenkins NA and Nagata S: The cDNA structure, expression, and

chromosomal assignment of the mouse Fas antigen. J Immunol 1992 (148):1274-1279

59 Rotello RJ, Liebermann RC, Purchio A and Gerschenson LE: Coordinated regulation of apoptosis and cell proliferation by transforming growth factor ß1 in cultured uterine epithelial cells. Proc Natl Acad Sci 1991 (88):3412-3415

60 Oberhammer F, Pavelka M, Sharma S, Tiefenbacher R, Purchio AF, Bursch W and Schulte-Hermann R: Induction of apoptosis in cultured hepatocytes and in regressing liver by transforming growth factor-ß1. Proc Natl Acad Sci USA 1992 (89):5408-5412

61 Bursch W, Oberhammer F, Jirtle RL, Askari M, Sedivy R, Grasl-Kraupp, Purchino AF and Schulte Hermann R: Transforming Growth Factor-ß1 as a signal for induction of cell death by apoptosis. Br J Cancer 1993 (67): 531-536

62 Massague J and Czech MP: The subunit structures of two distinct receptors for insulin-like growth factors I and II and their relationship to the insulin receptor. J Biol Chem 1982 (257):5038-5045

63 Scott CD and Baxter RC: Insulin-like growth factor-II receptors in cultured rat hepatocytes: regulation by cell density. J Cell Physiol 1987 (133):532-538

64 Lin JK and Chou CK: *In vitro* apoptosis in the human hepatoma cell line induced by transforming growth factor beta 1. Cancer Res 1992 (52):385-388

65 Yanagihara K and Tsumuraya M: Transforming growth factor beta 1 induces apoptotic cell death in cultured human gastric carcinoma cells. Cancer Res 1992 (52):4042-4045

66 Valverius EM, Walker-Jones D, Bates SE, Stampfer MR, Clark R, McCormick F, Dickson RB and Lippman ME: Production of and responsiveness to transforming growth factor-ß in normal and oncogene-transformed human mammary epithelial cells. Cancer Res 1989 (49):6269-6274

67 Thompson AM, Kerr DJ and Steel CM: Transforming growth factor ß1 is implicated in the failure of tamoxifen therapy in human breast cancer. Br J Cancer 1991 (63):609-614

68 Zugmaier G, Paik S, Wilding G, Knabbe C, Bano M, Lupu R, Deschauer B, Simpson S, Dickson R and Lippman M: Transforming growth factor ß1 induces cachexia and systemic fibrosis without an antitumor effect. Cancer Res 1991 (51):3590-3594

69 Evan GI, Wyllie AH, Gilbert CS, Littlewood TD, Land H, Brooks M, Waters CM, Penn LZ and Hancock DC: Induction of apoptosis in fibroblasts by c-*myc* protein. Cell 1992 (69):119-128

70 Shi Y, Glynn JM, Guilbert LJ, Cotter TG, Bissonnette RP and Green DR: Role of c-*myc* in activation-induced apoptotic cell death in T cell hybridomas. Science 1992 (257):212-214

71 Iseki R, Mukai M and Iwata M: Regulation of T lymphocyte apoptosis. Signals for the antagonism between activation- and glucocorticoid-induced death. J Immunol 1991 (147):4286-42922 56/290

72 Buttyan R, Olsson CA, Pintar J, Chang C, Bandyk M, Ng PY and Sawczuk IS: Induction of the TRPM-2 gene in cells undergoing programmed death. Mol Cell Biol 1989 (9):3473-3481

73 Colombel M, Olsson CA, Ng, PY and Buttyan R: Hormone-regulated apoptosis from reentry of differentiated prostate cells onto a defective cell cycle. Cancer Res 1992 (52): 4313-4319

74 Smyene RJ, Schilling K, Robertson L, Curran T and Morgan JI: *Fos-LacZ* transgenic mice: Mapping sites of gene induction in the central nervous system. Neuron 1992 (8):13-23

75 Hockenbery D, Zutter M, Hickey C, Nahm M and Korsmeyer SJ: *Bcl*-2 protein is topographically restricted in tissues characterized by apoptotic cell death. Proc Natl Acad Sci 1991 (88):6961-6965

76 Bissonette R, Echeverri F, Mahboubi A and Green D: Apoptotic cell death induced by c-*myc* is inhibited by *bcl*-2. Nature 1992 (359):552-554

77 Sentman CL, Shutter JR, Hockenbery D, Kanagawa O, Korsmeyer SJ: *bcl*-2 inhibits multiple forms of apoptosis but not negative selection in thymocytes. Cell 1991 (67):879-888

78 Teh BS, Chen P, Lavin MF, Seow WK and Thong YH: Demonstration of the induction of apoptosis (programmed cell death) by tetrandrine, a novel anti-inflammatory agent. Int J Immunopharmacol 1991 (13):1117-1126

79 Ellis RE, Yuan J and Horvitz HR: Mechanisms and functions of cell death. Annu Rev Cell Biol 1991 (7):663-698

80 Yonish-Rouach E, Resnitzky D, Lotem J, Sachs L, Kimchi A and Oren M: Wild-type *p53* induces apoptosis of myeloiod leukemia cells that is inhibited by interleukin-6. Nature 1991 (352):345-347

81 Bressac B, Kev M, Wands J and Ozturk M: Selective G to T mutations of *p53* gene in hepatocellular carcinoma from southern Africa. Nature 1991 (350):429-431

82 Zhang W, Hu G, Estey E; Hester J and Deisseroth A: Altered conformation of the *p53* protein in myeloid leukemia cells and mitogen-stimulated normal blood cells. Oncogene 1992 (7):1645-1647

83 Kastan MB, Onyekwere O, Sidransky D, Vogelstein B and Craig RW: Participation of *p53* protein in the cellular response to DNA damage. Cancer Res 1991 (51):6304-6311

84 Kuerbitz SJ, Plunkett BS, Walsh WV and Kastan MB: Wild-type is a cell cycle checkpoint determinant following irradiation. Proc Natl Acad Sci USA 1992 (89):7491-7495

85 Lane DP: *p53*, guardian of the genome. Nature 1992 (358):15-16

86 Yin Y, Tainsky MA, Bischoff FZ, Strong LC and Wahl GM: Wild-type *p53* restores cell cycle control and inhibits gene amplification in cells with mutant *p53* alleles. Cell 1992 (70):937-948

87 Shaw P, Bovey R, Tardy S, Sahli R, Sordat B, and Costa J: Induction of apoptosis by wild-type *p53* in a human colon tumor derived cell line. PNAS 1992 (89):4495-4499

88 Workman P, D'Incalci M, Berdel WE, Egorin MJ, Helene C, Hickman JA, Jarman M, Schwartsman G and Sikora K: New approaches in cancer pharmacology: Drug design and development. Eur J Cancer 1992 (28A):1190-1200

89 Bursch W, Fesus F and Schulte-Hermann R: Apoptosis ("programmed" cell death) and its

relevance in liver injury and carcinogenesis. In: Dekant W and Neumann HG (eds) Tissue Specific Toxicology. Academic Press, London 1992 pp 95-117

90 Ijiri K and Potten CS: Response of intestinal cells of differing topographical and hierarchical status to ten cytotoxic drugs and five sources of radiation. Br J Cancer 1983 (47):175-185

91 Lieberman MW, Verbin RS, Landay M, Liang H, Farber E, Lee T-N and Starr R: A probable role for protein synthesis in intestinal epithelial cell damage induced by cytosine arabinoside, nitrogen mustard, or X-irradiation. Cancer Res (30):942-951

92 Umansky SR, Korol BA and Nelipovich PA: *In vivo* DNA degradation in thymocytes of gamma-irradiated or hydrocortisone-treated rats. Biochim Biophys Acta 1981 (655):9-17

93 Mori N, Okumoto M, Morimoto J, Imai S, Matsuyama T, Takamori Y and Yagasaki O: Genetic analysis of susceptibility to radiation-induced apoptosis of thymocytes in mice. Int J Rad Biol 1992 (62):153-159

94 Warters,RL: Radiation-induced apoptosis in a murine T-cell hybridoma. Cancer Res 1992 (52):883-890

95 Eastman A: Activation of programmed cell death by anticancer agents: cisplatin as a model system. Cancer Cells 1990 (2):275-280

96 Grunicke H and Hofmann J: Cytotoxic and cytostatic effects of antitumor agents induced at the plasma membrane level. Pharmacol Therap 1993 (in press)

97 Cotter TG, Glynn JM, Echeverri F and Green DR: The induction of apoptosis by chemotherapeutic agents occurs in all phases of the cell cycle. Anticancer Res 1992 (12):773-779

98 Bruno S, Lassota P, Giratti W and Darzynkiewicz Z: Apoptosis of rat thymocytes triggered by prednisolone, camptothecin or teniposide is selective to G_0 cells and is prevented by inhibtors of proteases. Oncol Res 1992 (4):29-35

99 Dive C and Hickman JA: Drug-target interactions: only the first step in the commitment to a programmed cell death. Br J Cancer 1991 (64):192-196

100 Dive C, Evans CA and Whetton AD: Induction of apoptosis - New targets for cancer chemotherapy. Sem Cancer Biology 1992 (3):417-427

101 Baxter D and Lavin MF: Specific protein dephosphorylation in apoptosis induced by ionizing radiation and heat shock in human lymphoid tumor cell lines. J Immunol 1992 (148):1949-1954

102 Zubiaga AM, Munoz E and Huber BT: IL-4 and IL-2 selective rescue of Th cell subsets from glucocorticoid induced apoptosis. J Immunol 1992 (149):107-112

103 Rajotte D, Haddad P, Haman A, Cragoe EJ and Hoang T: Role of protein kinase C and the Na+H+ antiporter in suppression of apoptosis by granulocyte macrophage colony- stimulating factor and interleukin-3. Biol Chem 1992 (267):9980-9987

104 Ojeda F, Guarda MI, Maldonado C, Folch H and Diehl H: Role of protein kinase C in thymocyte apoptosis induced by irradiation. Int J Radiat Biol 1992 (61):663-667

105 Hickman JA: Membrane and signal transduction targets. In: Workman P (ed): New approaches in Cancer Pharmacology: Drug Design and Development. European School of Oncology Monographs. Springer Verlag, Heidelberg 1992 pp 33-46

106 Carson DA, Seto S, Wasson DB and Carrera CJ: DNA strand breaks, NAD metabolism, and programmed cell death, Exptl Cell Res 1986 (164):273-281

107 Wielckens K and Delfs T: Glucocorticoid-induced cell death and polyadenosine diphosphate (ADP) ribosylation: increased toxicity of dexamethasone on mouse S49.1 lymphoma cells with the poly(ADP-ribosyl)ation inhibitor benzamide. Endocrin 1986 (119):2383-2392

108 Hoshino J, Beckmann G and Kroger H: Sensitivity *in vitro* of mature mouse thymocytes to dexamethasone cytotoxicity and its correlation to poly ADP-ribosylation. Biochem Int 1992 (27):105-106

109 Marks DI and Fox RM: DNA damage, poly(ADP-ribosyl)ation and apoptotic cell death as potential common pathway of cytotoxic drug action. Biochem Pharmacol 1991 (42):1859-1867

110 Bertrand R, Sarang M, Jenkin J, Kerrigan D and Pommier Y: Differential induction of secondary DNA fragmentation by topoisomerase II inhibitors in human tumor cell lines with amplified *c-myc* expression. Cancer Res 1991 (51):6280-6285

111 Daoust R and Morais R: Degenerative changes, DNA synthesis and mitotic activity in rat liver following single exposure to diethylnitrosamine. Chem Biol Int 1986 (57):55-64

112 Wyllie AH: Apoptosis: cell death under homeostatic control. Arch Toxicol 1987 (Suppl 11): 3-10

113 Harmon BV, Corder AM, Collins RJ, Gobe GC, Allen J, Allan DJ and Kerr JFR: Cell death induced in a murine mastocytoma by 42 to 47°C heating *in vitro*: evidence that the form of death changes from apoptosis to necrosis above a critical heat load. Int J Radiat Biol 1990 (58):845-858

114 Soloff BL, Nagle WA, Moss AJ, Henle KJ and Crawford JT: Apoptosis induced by cold shock *in vitro* is dependent on cell growth phase. Biochem Biophys Res Comm 1987 (145):876-883

115 Gorczyca W, Bruno S, Melamed MR and Darzynkiewicz Z: Cell cycle-related expression of p120 nulear antigen in normal human lymphocytes and in cells of HL-60 and MOLT-4 leukemic lines: effect of methotrexate, camptothecin and teniposide. Cancer Res 1992 (52):3491-3494

116 Bursch W, Paffe S, Putz B, Barthel G and Schulte-Hermann R: Determination of the length of the histological stages of apoptosis in normal liver and in altered hepatic foci of rats. Carcinogenesis 1990 (11):847-853

117 Potten CS, Al-Barwari SE and Searle J: Differential radiation response amongst proliferating epithelial cells. Cell Tiss Kin 1978 (11): 149-169

118 Arends MJ, Morris RG and Wyllie AH: Apoptosis - The role of endonuclease. Am J Pathol 1990 (136):593-607

119 Cohen GM, Sun XM, Snowden RT, Dinsdale D and Skileter DN: Key morphological features of apoptosis may occur in the absence of

internucleosomal DNA fragmentation. Biochem J 1992 (286):331-334

120 Oberhammer F, Fritsch G, Schmied M, Pavelka M, Printz D, Purchio T, Lassmann H and Schulte-Hermann R: Condensation of the chromatin at the membrane of an apoptotic nucleus is not associated with activation of an endonuclease. J Cell Science 1993 (104): 317-326

121 Collins RJ, Harmon V, Gobé GC and Kerr JFR: Internucleosomal DNA cleavage should not be the sole criterion for identifying apoptosis. Int J Radiat Biol 1992 (61):451-453

122 Martz E and Howell DM: CTL: Virus control cells first and cytoloytic cells second? DNA fragmentation, apoptosis and the prelytic halt hypothesis. Immunol Today 1989 (10):79-86

123 Fesus L, Davies PJ and Piacentini M: Apoptosis: molecular mechanisms in programmed cell death. Eur J Cell Biol 1991 (56):107-117

124 Bursch W, Kleine L and Tenniswood MP: The biochemistry of cell death by apoptosis. Biochem Cell Biol 1990 (68):1071-1074

125 Clarke PH: Developmental cell death: morphological diversity and multiple mechanisms. Anat Embryol 1990 (181):195-213

Engineering Antibodies for Targeted Cancer Therapy

Robert E. Hawkins

MRC Laboratory of Molecular Biology, Hills Road, Cambridge CB2 2HQ, United Kingdom

The last few years have seen a revolution in molecular biology which has allowed greater understanding of the mechanisms of oncogenesis. Unfortunately this greater understanding has not yet led to improved therapy. However, these same techniques are now being applied to developing new therapeutic modalities. Antibodies are flexible binding reagents and are being investigated as tumour targeting agents. Recently the development of new methods has allowed improved antibodies to be made. Equally importantly, the use of genetic engineering allows novel therapeutic molecules, based on antibodies, to be prepared. In addition, antibodies will play a part in many other approaches to targeted cancer therapy including gene therapy and the development of cancer vaccines. The next few years will increasingly see the application of molecular biology to the therapy of human disease and in particular the therapy of cancer.

Experience of Antibody Targeted Cancer Therapy

Since the development of monoclonal antibodies by somatic cell fusion [1], numerous antibodies to (relatively) tumour-specific antigens have been made. They provide useful diagnostic (for review see [2]) and prognostic [3] information in the treatment of cancer and have been tested for imaging or therapy in a variety of malignancies. In general, imaging is successful, although probably little better than other available techniques, but therapeutic successes have been limited (for review see [4]). The reasons for this are illustrated in Table 1.

Many of these problems are interrelated. Poor penetration, poor target specificity and lower than optimal affinity mean that only a small fraction of the antibody reaches the tumour (usually much less than 1%) and that it frequently localises only around the tumour vasculature. Because many antibodies have poor affinity they remain bound for only a short time. A humanised antibody has been used with good effect in the treatment of non-Hodgkin's lymphoma [5] but for common epithelial tumours, the use of optimal (i.e., full human or humanised) antibodies has not been reported. The use of natural effector mechanisms remains attractive both because they should have low toxicity and because the mechanism of action is entirely different to that of radiation or cytotoxic drugs. Antibody-guided radiation, most commonly radio-iodine, has been used extensively as an alternative. This has the advan-

Table 1. Problems encountered in antibody therapy for cancer

- Poor specificity of target antigens

- Heterogeneous expression of target antigens

- Poor penetration of solid tumours by large molecules

- Antibodies used may have suboptimal affinity

- Immunogenicity of the antibody limits long-term therapy

- Toxicity resulting from the effector arm of the antibody

Table 2. Target antigens for anticancer MAbs

• Unique to tumour	Immunoglobulins T cell receptors Mutated cell surface proteins
• Relative abundance in tumour	Growth factor receptors Oncofetal antigens Dead cell markers Altered carbohydrate groups
• Confined to tumour and nonessential normal tissues	Differentiation antigens
• Stromal targets	Endothelial activation markers Fibroblast activation markers

tage that part of the problem of tumour penetration is overcome but the low percentage of the dose received and the extensive circulation time mean that much of the radiation dose is received by other tissues, including very sensitive tissues such as bone marrow. Overall, even though responses can be achieved in very radiosensitive tumours [6], there may be considerable toxicity. Understanding the problems involved and applying the techniques of molecular biology to solving them should allow new molecules, which overcome at least some of these problems, to be made. This chapter will examine some of these problems, new ways of making antibodies, ways of expressing antibodies to allow their optimal use for therapy and the application of antibodies in other approaches to targeted cancer therapy.

Target Antigens

There are a number of classes of tumour antigens (Table 2). The main target antigens used in human trials have been over-expressed oncofetal antigens or differentiation markers. In nude mouse models such antigens generally provide excellent targets but in humans the targeting ability is often less impressive. There may be many reasons for this but part of the problem is the presence of the identical or cross-reactive antigens in normal tissues. Even weakly cross-reactive tissue may be important

[7] especially if it is more accessible as the amount bound is very dependent on the amount reaching the target [8]. Such cross-reactivities have occasionally given rise to unexpected toxicities in human trials [7]. Intensive effort has, however, revealed some tumour-specific mutant cell-surface proteins; they deserve special note both because they make ideal targets and because further such markers may be discovered. Such markers have been encountered as a result of point mutation (e.g., Her 2 in breast cancer), deletion (e.g., mutant EGF receptors encountered in malignant gliomas) and chromosome translocation (tropomysin-tyrosine kinase fusion in colon carcinoma) (for review see [9]).

Contrary to the popular view of cancer, one feature which characterises many tumours is the increased cell death. This exposes markers not found in normal tissues and they are thus potentially useful therapeutic targets if used in conjunction with effector mechanisms which have appropriate bystander effects [10]. Stromal and endothelial activation markers could similarly provide general tumour targets. Although certainly not ideal for eradicating all microscopic disease, such an approach coupled to appropriate effector mechanisms may be a very effective and general approach for targeting bulk disease.

Advances in our understanding of carbohydrate metabolism and carbohydrate chemistry have led to the discovery that many tumours contain an abundance of altered carbohydrates [11]. In some cases this involves glycolipids as well as glycoproteins, making these especially abundant targets. In addition, there is increasing evidence that such carbohydrate groups are involved as adhesion molecules and in the development of metastasis [12]. Their presence is correlated with poor prognosis [13,14]. Targeted therapy against such molecules is therefore especially attractive.

Tumour Penetration by Macromolecules

Our understanding of tumour vasculature and the penetration of macromolecules into solid tumours is incomplete but some principles are clear. Studies with various high molecular weight dextrans demonstrate that the tumour neovasculature is more permeable than normal blood vessels and this allows the leakage of macromolecules from the vessels [15,16]. However, once extravasated they penetrate the tumour parenchyma slowly and inefficiently. This applies to antibodies and must clearly be considered when designing targeting molecules.

Binding Characteristics - Affinity and Avidity

The antibody binding to its antigen is clearly important. As indicated above, the specificity is one aspect but for optimal targeting the affinity of binding is also important. The antibody interaction with its antigen is usually described by its affinity but this is actually a composite of the kinetic "on-rate" and "off-rate". The antigen targets usually have relatively high concentrations and as the speed of diffusion through the tumour is slow there is plenty of time for binding to occur. The targeting is therefore more determined by the rate of dissociation from the tumour in relation to the rate of blood clearance. One major determinant of this is the "off-rate" of the antibody (see below).

In addition to affinity and off-rate there are other features of binding which can be used to advantage. Natural antibodies are (at least) bivalent and use this feature to improve binding. The affinity of binding results from univalent interactions but when binding of two or more heads occurs this results in a much more stable interaction - known as the avidity effect. This can result in large increases in functional affinity (up to 1000-fold for an IgG compared to an Fab) but depends critically on the density of the target antigen in relation to the spacing of the antibody heads [17]. Whole antibodies use this feature but by careful design it may be possible to make molecules that are small and thus penetrate well but are avid and so bind strongly (see below).

Immunogenicity

Rodent antibodies are immunogenic in humans resulting in progressively shorter half-life of injected antibody with repeated dosage. Although rare in practice, this can also result in toxic side effects such as serum sickness or anaphylaxis. Production of chimeric [18] or fully reshaped antibodies [19] allows this problem

Table 3. The ideal targeting reagent

- Small - preferably less than 40 kDa

- Bind with high affinity

- Human

- Non-toxic before bound

- Effector mechanism should amplify the amount bound

- Effector mechanism should have bystander effect

---

to be reduced or avoided but rapid methods of making human antibodies directly are desirable.

Engineering Improved Antibodies for Therapy

The problems outlined above suggest that the ideal targeting reagent (Table 3) would be small (say <40,000 Da), have high affinity and slow off-rate from its antigen (either intrinsically or by making use of avidity effects). The molecule should be seen as human by the immune system to avoid immune responses. Nevertheless, the experience to date suggests that the amount of targeted reagent reaching the tumour will remain low in terms of % injected dose/gram tumour. This implies that the preferred effector mechanism should incorporate some amplification and should be non-toxic in the delivered form. In addition, tumour antigen heterogeneity and the difficulty of reaching all cells suggest that the effector end of the molecule should have bystander effects. The extent to which the genetic manipulation of antibodies will allow us to approach this ideal is discussed below.

New Methods of Making Antibodies - the Phage System

Since an antibody fragment was first expressed on the surface of bacteriophage [20], rapid development of this approach to making antibodies has occurred. This system has 4 major advantages over other existing methods for making antibodies (Table 4).

Table 4. Advantages in using phage to make antibodies for therapy

---

- Human antibodies can be made directly

- Large numbers of antibodies can be made

- Selection for high affinity (and slow off-rate) is possible

- The antibody genes are obtained directly allowing expression in many different forms

---

The basic technology behind the use of phage to make antibodies is the polymerase chain reaction (PCR). Using suitable primers [21], PCR can be used to amplify repertoires of re-arranged V-genes [22] from a variety of B-cell subsets [23]. Once amplified, these gene libraries can be joined together as an antibody fragment and cloned into phage expression vectors. The display of antibodies on the surface of phage means that the phage can be treated exactly as if it were an antibody and thus selected for specificity and desired binding characteristics [24]. After the initial selection, various methods of mutagenesis can be used to improve the originally selected antibodies [25,26]. In fact, the whole process has many similarities to the humoral immune system. By using repertoires from non-immune humans [27], we can make and affinity mature human antibodies to many different antigens just as in the natural immune system (Fig. 1). The process of making phage antibodies is rapid and more efficient than cell immortalisation and thus allows many different antibodies to any given antigen to be produced. As polyclonal antisera have been shown to be more effective than monoclonal antibodies in the treatment of recurrent Hodgkin's disease with radiolabelled anti-ferritin antibodies [6], it may be that the use of monoclonal cocktails will improve on single antibodies. Indeed, it may be expected that, in view of tumour antigen heterogeneity, the use of multiple antibodies to multiple antigens will be more effective still.

As suggested above, specificity, affinity and off-rate are important features of an antibody. Recent evidence suggests that, in an animal model, the use of higher affinity antibodies leads to improved anti-tumour activity and improved survival [28]. The use of the bacteriophage system allows the initial selection of antibody by affinity and also allows the improvement of existing antibodies [25].

The final advantage of the phage system is that it permits the selection of antibodies as cloned DNA which can very easily be expressed in an ever increasing number of ways. This facilitates the attachment of many novel effector mechanisms and even the direct use of *in vivo* gene expression to deliver the therapeutic antibody.

New Molecules for Antibody-Targeted Cancer Therapy

Genetic manipulation allows the production of an endless variety of antibody-derived molecules. The basic types are shown in Figure 2. The ideal therapeutic agent does not exist but developments of new reagents that

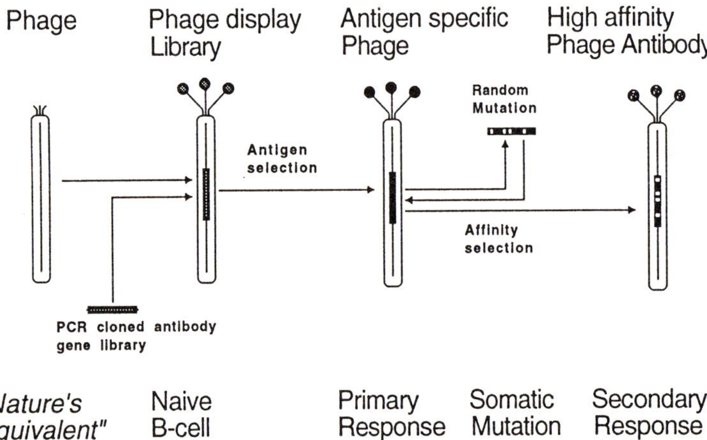

Fig. 1. Comparison of the phage system for making antibodies from natural libraries with the immune system. The initial large repertoire of scFv fragments is equivalent to the naive B-cell repertoire and amongst this repertoire antibodies can be found to any antigen. The affinity can subsequently be improved using methods of mutagenesis and phage selection.

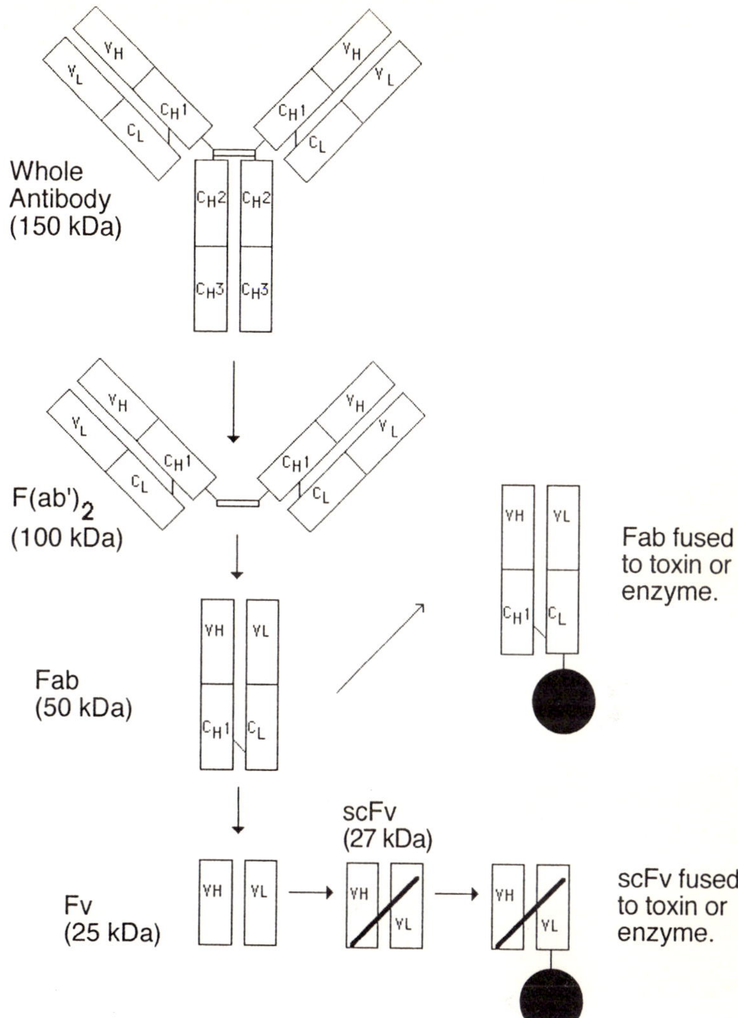

Fig. 2. The various formats of antibodies used for therapy with their molecular weight. The size is important for tumour penetration and is also an important determinant of the circulating half-life. The Fab and scFv can also be produced as bispecific antibodies. These fragments can be produced in eukaryotic cells or bacteria.

fulfil at least some of the criteria for an ideal molecule (Table 3) have been reported.

Improving Tumour Penetration

Two approaches that have been investigated to improve tumour penetration are antibody-interleukin-2 conjugates which appear to increase the local vascular permeability [29] or the use of small antibody fragments. It has been shown that scFv versions of antibodies (MW = 27,000) permeate deep into the tumour after 30 minutes whereas it takes 24 hours or more for a whole IgG molecule (MW 150,000) to achieve comparable penetration [30]. Even then, the penetration of IgG at distances greater than 50 mm from the blood vessel is less than that for a scFv. These are important considerations for tumour targeting and when choosing the optimal effector mechanism. The

use of antibody engineering to produce a scFv-IL2 fusion would combine these approaches.

Although allowing better penetration, the small size of the scFv means that it is rapidly cleared through the kidneys and thus has a short serum half-life [31]. In addition, it is univalent and so must rely on intrinsic affinity rather than avidity to remain bound in the tumour. Nevertheless, an unmodified form of the scFv may be used as a convenient imaging reagent since images can be obtained within hours rather than the days required for whole antibodies [32]. For therapy, radiation is the only effector function that can be used without increasing the size of the molecule, but the short blood half-life means that only a low fraction of the dose will reach the tumour. These molecules are, however, being engineered to modify these characteristics. Bivalent single chain Fv molecules can be made using tags of amphipathic helices that are covalently associated or in dynamic equilibrium with the monomer [33]. Such molecules overcome the loss of avidity, may have longer circulation time and yet still be able to penetrate the tumour well. An extension of this approach could use different dimerising tags which preferentially form heterodimers [34]. The use of such antibodies binding two different target molecules would simultaneously increase both avidity and specificity. If the two antibodies are not covalently associated but dimerise with appropriate affinity, it may even be possible to build up larger molecules within the tumour from small ones in the circulation. Because the small molecules penetrate well, the amount reaching deep into the tumour is relatively large. Once a critical concentration is reached, dimerisation to form a bivalent molecule will occur rendering the binding more stable by virtue of the functional avidity.

Cell Killing Mechanisms

A variety of cell killing mechanisms have been linked to antibodies in addition to their natural effector mechanisms. They are summarised in Table 5. The effector mechanisms that will probably benefit most from the ability to engineer antibodies are the use of natural immunological mechanisms of cell killing and the antibody-directed enzyme prodrug therapy (ADEPT) approach. Radiation has been used extensively and new isotopes that may have improved characteristics are being investigated [35], but the basic problem is to target a sufficient dose to the tumour without systemic toxicity - improved antibody design may make this possible for the more radiation-sensitive tumours, but for others large improvements are needed. Similarly, although the development of toxins is facilitated by new protein engineering constructs [36], the problems of tumour antigen heterogeneity and tumour penetration to reach all cells remain. For drug conjugates there is a further problem of getting sufficient drug to the target. This may be improved by the use of more potent drugs. Thus, although suitable combinations of such reagents may be useful, other options are more attractive.

Initial trials of a fully humanised antibody in non-Hodgkin's lymphoma gave encouraging remissions [5] but until recently human antibodies to common epithelial tumour antigens were not available. The widespread use of humani-

Table 5. Comparison of antibody effector mechanisms

FEATURE	EFFECTOR MECHANISM				
	Natural antibody	Radiation	Toxin conjugate	Drug conjugate	ADEPT
Minimum size[a]	150 kDa	25 kDa	65 kDa	25 kDa	<1 kDa
Bystander effects	Yes	Yes	No	No	Yes
Immunogenic	No	No[b]	Yes[c]	No	Yes[c]
Toxicity of unbound form	Low	High	Low[d]	Low[d]	Low[e]
Amplifies signal	Yes	No	No	No	Yes

All antibody components are human or humanised.
a   Penetration of large tumours is largely a function of the size of the molecule. It is certainly poor for any molecule of 40 kDa or more.
b   Antibody responses can occur to the chelating agent when this method of coupling radiation is used.
c   Current constructs involve toxins/enzymes that are non-human and thus immunogenic but newer forms may be made from human proteins and thus be non-antigenic.
d   Toxicity partly depends on the method of linkage used. In vivo instability has been a problem with some methods. For toxins this can be overcome by using fusion proteins.
e   The toxicity depends on the prodrug. There may be some activation of drugs in normal tissues and thus some toxicity.

sation [37] and direct production using phage antibodies [27] is changing this. The use of human antibodies has the advantage that they should (especially if used as appropriate cocktails) be relatively non-toxic. Their use, perhaps over prolonged periods, may well be effective where rodent antibodies, which suffer the twin disadvantages of poor recruitment of effector mechanisms and immunogenicity, were not.

Other ways of recruiting natural effector mechanisms are increasingly being investigated and may be advantageous. In particular various methods are being employed to direct and activate T-cells using antibodies. These include the use of bispecific antibodies to recruit effector cells [38]. Such molecules have been administered with good effect in the treatment of malignant glioma [39] and the new methods of producing bispecific antibodies [34,40] will enable their more widespread application. A final interesting alternative approach to harness cell-mediated immunity is the use of powerful T-cell activators, such as superantigens, linked to antibodies [41]. Such natural mechanisms may be used alone, in combination with cytokines and perhaps with adoptive immunotherapy [42] to further stimulate the anti-tumour response.

Of the artificial effector mechanisms the ADEPT system [43] is attractive. In this approach an antibody is used to target an enzyme to the tumour and retain it there while the conjugate clears from the circulation. At this stage a non-toxic prodrug is given which is activated by the enzyme to produce a cytotoxic drug. This system has the attractions that it includes an element of amplification and that the final cytotoxic molecule is small, allowing diffusion throughout the tumour. Thus, it is unnecessary to reach all the cells and activation of the prodrug in the vicinity of the tumour may be sufficient. The obvious drawback is the need to develop appropriate drug/antibody-enzyme combinations. Nevertheless, such reagents are being reported. The ideal approach has not yet been found but the expression of human ß-glucuronidase as an antibody fusion product [44] is the only report of an entirely human construct. Appropriate drugs are not yet widely available but preliminary tests with epirubicin glucuronide as the prodrug appear promising [45] and nitrogen mustard glucuronides [46] are further possibilities.

Antibodies and Other Approaches to Targeted Cancer Therapy

Other techniques are emerging which use antibodies as a major part of the mechanism of tumour targeting. Methods of developing cancer vaccines and gene therapy are particularly noteworthy.

Cancer Vaccines

Breaking host tolerance towards tumours is attractive and methods of immunisation aimed at doing this are being developed. Many of these are based on the use of recombinant viruses, especially vaccinia virus [47]. As mentioned above (Table 2), there are a few truly tumour-specific markers; these make ideal targets for antibody therapy and they are also attractive targets for the induction of active immunity. The attraction of the vaccine approach is that the protection should be present on a continuing basis. In addition, T-cell immunity as well as an antibody response can be induced and this should improve the level of protection. The prototype tumour-specific target is the idiotypic immunoglobulin expressed on B-cell malignancies. Although anti-idiotype antibodies have achieved prolonged remissions in a few patients [48], the difficulty of making monoclonal antibodies on an individual patient basis has limited their use. The alternative approach of immunising patients with the idiotypic immunoglobulin is attractive and preliminary results seem promising [49], but there are still considerable problems in producing such vaccines on an individual basis. The direct use of PCR to clone the antibody genes from tumour biopsies is a more rapid way of identifying the idiotypic immunoglobulin which acts as the immunogen [50]. Furthermore, the recently described process of genetic immunisation [51] simplifies the process of producing a vaccine on an individual patient basis. In this procedure the proposed immunogen is cloned into a eukaryotic expression vector, DNA is prepared and directly injected. Once injected, some of the DNA is taken up by cells, expressed and an immune response made. This very simple procedure can be adapted to made anti-idiotypic vaccines [50] but should also be a simple way of making vaccines to multiple tumour antigens identified in an individual patient's tumour. The advantage of this system, in addition to its simplicity, is that it mimics viral vaccines which are known to be highly effective and yet it is not replicating and so has fewer risks. As more tumour-specific antigens are discovered [9], extension to other tumours will be possible. In particular, if cytotoxic T-cell responses can be generated [52], then the use of intracellular antigens as targets will be possible. Particularly attractive intracellular targets are mutant forms of p53 or ras. Animal experiments and the initial clinical data [49] suggest that this form of therapy will be most effective in patients with limited disease, so it will be most likely to be used as a adjunct to other therapy.

Gene Therapy

Using Genes to Deliver Antibodies

Gene therapy is likely to be a major area in cancer therapy in its own right but cross-fertilisation with developments in antibody therapy will occur. One of the drawbacks of protein therapy of all types is the difficulty and cost of making and testing large quantities of the therapeutic molecule. The rapid progress with methods of bacterial expression [40,53] alleviate this problem, but certainly from a practical point of view the use of gene transfer as a means of producing antibodies is attractive. The permanent production of proteins required for corrective gene therapy requires stable integration of genes and is perhaps best achieved using viruses (e.g. retroviruses or adeno-associated viruses). However, for therapy with antibodies or any of the derivatives mentioned above, short-term production is all that is required. Currently, adenoviruses are being evaluated for delivery of therapeutic proteins and are flexible vectors for gene transfer which allow the incorporation of relatively large amounts of foreign DNA [54]. However, for such treatment the immunogenicity of viruses is likely to compromise repeated therapy. A plethora of other methods available for *in vivo* gene transfer include liposomes, protein-coupled DNA or even direct injection of DNA (for review see [55]). Such methods of gene transfer are currently rather inefficient but by incorporating the relevant parts of viral coat proteins into the DNA-protein complex the efficiency of DNA entry into the cell is improved [56]. Further improvements to these approaches may make repeated therapy possible and enable the efficient *in vivo* production of any therapeutic proteins including antibodies.

Using Antibodies to Deliver Genes

Direct expression of an appropriate toxin within the tumour itself is perhaps an ideal. For this, targeted delivery of genetic information is needed. One approach is the use of antibodies to target the genes. Antibodies can be employed to target liposomes [57], viruses [58] or even directly to target DNA for gene delivery to specific tissues [59]. The size of such particles means that access to tumour tissues is severely limited. Here, if safe replication competent viral vectors can be developed, viruses have the decisive advantage that they can replicate; one infected cell will produce not only many molecules of the therapeutic agent but also many progeny viruses which can infect more cells by local spread. In this regard, the preliminary report of stable incorporation of a functional antibody into the envelope protein of a retrovirus is exciting [60]. If the viral infection can be directed by the antibody then it would allow targeted DNA delivery. Even without this feature the antibody would retain the virus on antigen-positive cells. Thus some degree of targeting will be achievable and should be valuable in terms of both safety and efficacy. Certainly there are problems of efficient gene transfer and problems of immunogenicity, but in time, if these can be overcome or circumvented, such recombinant viruses could provide an efficient means of reaching large tumour deposits.

Conclusion

Molecular biology is rapidly changing antibody-targeted therapy. Firstly, new targets are being discovered. Secondly, it has led to the development of new methods of making antibodies which should be superior to the cell-based methods. Thirdly, the antibodies can be expressed in many forms with many different effector molecules. The most important advances are likely to be from the use of small fragments, from improved methods of recruiting natural effector mechanisms and from targeting enzymes to activate prodrugs. Indeed these methods may be especially effective if used together. The ADEPT system should be very effective but the problem of drug resistance in a small proportion of the tumour will be an ever present problem. Nevertheless, at the very least, we can expect to reduce drug toxicity by such an approach. By contrast, the strength of natural mechanisms of immune surveillance is their low toxicity and entirely different mode of action. The use of true human antibodies or true human bispecific antibodies may allow prolonged therapy. This may be augmented by stimulation of T-cell immunity either with cytokines, by adoptive immunotherapy, or by using immunisation with tumour-specific antigens to stimulate the immune system. Such combined approaches should be very effective at directing the immune system to eradicate or suppress residual disease. Finally, gene therapy techniques for the treatment of cancer are making rapid progress. Antibodies may either be used to target appropriate genes or the appropriate vectors may be used to allow *in vivo* production of antibody-based molecules.

There are now a plethora of new techniques available which will allow us to test therapeutic modalities, involving the use of antibodies, for the targeted therapy of cancer. It is certain that all possible permutations cannot be tested and perhaps the main need now is to apply our knowledge of the principles involved to design suitable molecules and test them in appropriate clinical settings.

REFERENCES

1   Kohler G and Milstein C: Continuous cultures of fused cells secreting antibody of predefined specificity. Nature 1975 (256):495-497
2   Neville AM: Detection of tumor antigens with monoclonal antibodies: immunopathology and immunodiagnosis. Curr Opin Immunol 1991 (3):674-678
3   Hawkins RE, Roberts K, Wiltshaw E, Mundy J, Fryatt IJ and McCready VR: The prognostic significance of the half-life of serum CA125 in patients responding to chemotherapy for epithelial ovarian carcinoma. Br J Obstet Gynaecol 1989 (96):1395-1399
4   Mach J-P, Pelegrin A and Buchegger F: Imaging and therapy with monoclonal antibodies in non-hematopoietic tumors. Curr Opin Immunol 1991 (3):685-693
5   Hale G, Clark MR, Marcus R, Winter G, Dyer MJS, Phillips JM, Riechmann L and Waldmann H: Remission induction in non-Hodgkin lymphoma with reshaped monoclonal antibody CAMPATH-1H. Lancet 1988 (ii): 1394-1399
6   Vriesendorp HM, Herpst JM, Germack MA, Klein JL, Leichner PK, Loudenslager DM, et al: Phase I-II studies of yttrium-labelled antiferritin treatment for end-stage Hodgkin's disease, including radiation therapy oncology group 87-01. J Clin Oncol 1991 (9):918-928
7   Pai LH, Bookman MA, Ozols RF, Young RC, Smith JW, Longo DL, Gould B, Frankel A, McClay EF, Howell S, Reed E, Willingham MC, Fitzgerald DJ and Pastan I: Clinical evaluation of intraperitoneal pseudomonas exotoxin immunoconjugate OVB3-PE in patients with ovarian cancer. J Clin Oncol 1991 (9): 2095-2103
8   Kennel SJ: Effects of target antigen competition on distribution of monoclonal antibody to solid tumors. Cancer Res 1991 (52):1284-1290
9   Urban JL and Schreiber H: Tumor antigens. Annu Rev Immunol 1992 (10):617-644
10 Epstein AL, Chen FM and Taylor CR: A novel method for the detection of necrotic lesions in human cancers. Cancer Res 1988 (48):5842-5848
11 Hakomori S: Aberrant glycosylation in tumors and tumor-associated carbohydrate antigens. Adv Cancer Res 1989 (52): 257-331
12 Hoff SD, Irimura T, Matsushita Y, Ota DM, Cleary KR and Hakomori S: Metastatic potential of colon carcinoma: expression of ABO/Lewis-realted antigens. Arch Surg 1990 (125):206-209
13 Hakomori S: Possible functions of tumor-associated carbohydrate antigens. Curr Opin Immunol 1991 (3): 646-653
14 Itzkowitz SH, Bloom EJ, Kokai WA, Modin G, Hakomori S and Kim YS: Sialosyl-Tn: a novel mucin antigen associated with prognosis in colorectal cancer patients. Cancer 1990 (66): 1960-1966
15 Dvorak HF, Nagy JA and Dvorak AM: Structure of solid tumors and their vasculature: Implications for therapy with monoclonal antibodies. Cancer Cells 1991 (3):77-85
16 Dvorak HF, Nagy JA, Dvorak JT and Dvorak AM: Identification and characterization of the blood vessels of solid tumors that are leaky to circulating macromolecules. Am J Pathol 1988 (133): 95-109
17 Kaufman EN and Jain RK: Effect of bivalent interaction upon apparent antibody affinity: experimental confirmation of a theory using fluorescence photobleaching and implications for antibody binding assays. Cancer Res. 1992 (52): 4157-4167
18 Neuberger MS, Williams GT, Mitchell EB, Jouhal SS, Flanagan, JG and Rabbitts TH: A hapten-specific chimaeric IgE with human physiological effector function. Nature (Lond.) 1985 (314): 268-270
19 Riechmann L, Clark M, Waldmann H and Winter G: Reshaping human antibodies for therapy. Nature 1988 (332):323-327
20 McCafferty J, Griffiths AD, Winter G and Chiswell DJ: Phage antibodies: filamentous phage displaying antibody variable domains. Nature (London) 1990 (348):552-554
21 Orlandi R, Güssow DH, Jones PT and Winter G: Cloning immunoglobulin variable domains for expression by the polymerase chain reaction. Proc Natl Acad Sci USA 1989 (86):3833-3837
22 Ward ES, Güssow D, Griffiths AD, Jones PT and Winter G: Binding activities of a repertoire of single immunoglobulin variable domains secreted from *Escherichia coli*. Nature (London) 1989 (344):544-546
23 Hawkins RE and Winter G: Cell selection strategies for making antibodies from variable gene libraries: tapping the memory pool. Eur J Immunol 1992 (22):867-870
24 Clackson T, Hoogenboom HR, Griffiths AD and Winter G: Making antibody fragments using phage display libraries. Nature (London) 1991 (352):624-628
25 Hawkins RE, Russell SJ and Winter G: Selection of phage antibodies by binding affinity: mimicking affinity maturation. J Mol Biol 1992 (226):889-896
26 Marks JD, Griffiths AD, Malmqvist M, Clackson TP, Bye JM and Winter G: By-passing immunisation: improving the affinity of a human antibody by chain shuffling. Bio/Technology 1992 (10):779-783
27 Marks JD, Hoogenboom HR, Bonnert TP, MacCafferty J, Griffiths AD: By-passing immunization: human antibodies from V-gene libraries displayed on bacteriophage. J Mol Biol 1991 (222):581-597
28 Schlom J, Eggensperger D, Colcher D, Molinolo A, Houchens D, Miller LS, Hinkle G and Siler K: Therapeutic advantage of high-affinity anticarcinoma radioimmunoconjugates. Cancer Res 1992 (52): 1067-1072
29 LeBerthon B, Khawli LA, Alaudin M, Miller GK, Charak BS, Mazumder A and Epstein AL: Enhanced tumor uptake of macromolecules induced by a novel vasoactive interleukin 2 immunoconjugate. Cancer Res 1991 (51):2694-2698
30 Yokata T, Milenic DE, Whitlow M and Schlom J: Rapid tumor penetration of a single-chain Fv and comparison with other immunoglobulin forms. Cancer Res 1992 (52):3402-3408

31 Milenic DE, Yokota T, Filpula DR, Finkelman MAJ, Dodd SW, Wood JF et al: Construction, binding properties, metabolism, and tumor targeting of a single-chain Fv derived from the pancarcinoma monoclonal antibody CC49. Cancer Res 1991 (51):6363-6371

32 Colcher D, Bird R, Roselli M, Hardman KD, Johnson S, Pope S, Dodd SW, Pantoliano MW, Milenic DE and Schlom J: In vivo tumor targeting of a recombinant single-chain antigen binding protein. JNCI 1990 (82):1191-1197

33 Pack P and Plückthun A: Miniantibodies: use of amphipathic helices to produce functional, flexibly linked dimeric Fv fragments with high avidity in *Escherichia coli*. Biochemistry 1992 (31):1579-1584

34 Kostelny SA, Cole MS and Tso JY: Formation of a bispecific antibody by use of leucine zippers. J Immunol 1992 (148):1547-1553

35 Waldmann TA: Monoclonal antibodies in diagnosis and therapy. Science 1991 (252):1657-1662

36 Rybak SM, Hoogenboom HR, Meade HM, Raus JCM, Schwartz D and Youle RJ: Humanization of immunotoxins. Proc Natl Acad Sci USA 1992 (89):3165-3169

37 Carter P, Presa L, Gorman CM, Ridgway JBB, Henner D, Wong WLT, Rowland AM, Kotts C, Carver ME and Shepard HM: Humanisation of an anti-p185^{HER2} antibody for human cancer therapy. Proc Natl Acad Sci USA 1992 (89) 4285-4289

38 Staerz UD, Kanagawa O and Bevan MJ: Hybrid antibodies can target sites for attack by T-cells. Nature 1985 (314): 628-631

39 Nitta T, Sato K, Yagita H, Okumura K and Ishii S: Preliminary trial of specific targeting therapy against malignant glioma. Lancet 1990 (335):368-371

40 Carter P, Kelley RF, Rodrigues ML, Snedecor B, Covarrubias Velligan MD, Wong WLT, Rowland, AM, Kotts CE, Carver ME, Yang M, Bourell JH, Shephard HM and Henner D: High level *Escherichia coli* expression and production of bivalent humanized antibody fragment. Bio/technology 1992 (10): 163-167

41 Dohlestein M, Hedlund G, Åkerblom E, Lando PA and Kalland T: Monoclonal antibody-targeted super-antigens: a different class of anti-tumor agents. Proc Natl Acad Sci USA 1991 (88): 9287-9291

42 Rosenburg SA: The immunotherapy and gene therapy of cancer. J Clin Oncol 1992 (10):180-199

43 Bagshaw KD: Towards generating cytotoxic agents at cancer sites. Br J Cancer 1989 (60):275-281

44 Bosslet K, Czech J, Lorenz P, Sedlacek HH, Schuermann M and Seeman G: Molecular and functional characterisation of a fusion protein suited for tumour specific prodrug activation. Br J Cancer 1992 (65):234-238

45 Haisma HJ, Boven E, van Muijen M, de Jong J, van der Vijgh WJ and Pinedo HM: A monoclonal antibody-ß-glucuronidase conjugate as activator of the prodrug epirubicin-glucuronide for specific treatment of cancer. Br J Cancer 1992 (66):474-478

46 Wang S-M, Chern J-W, Yeh M-W, Ng JC, Tung E and Roffler SR: Specific activation of glucuronide prodrugs by antibody-targeted enzyme conjugates for cancer therapy. Cancer Res 1992 (52):4484-4491

47 Hareuveni M, Gautier C, Kieny M-P, Wreschner D, Chambon P, Lathe R: Vaccination against tumour cells expressing breast cancer epithelial tumor antigen. Proc Natl Acad Sci USA 1990 (87): 9498-9502

48 Miller RA, Maloney DG, Warnke R and Levy R: Treatment of B-cell lymphoma with monoclonal anti-idiotype antibody. N Engl J Med 1982 (306):517-522

49 Kwak LW, Campbell MJ, Czerwinski DK, Hart S, Miller RA and Levy R: Induction of immune responses in patients with B-cell lymphoma against the surface-imunoglobulin idiotype expressed by their tumours. N Engl J Med 1992 (327):1209-1215

50 Hawkins RE, Winter G, Hamblin TJ, Stevenson F and Russell SJ: A genetic approach to idiotype vaccination. J Immunother 1993 (in press)

51 Tang D-C, DeVit M, Johnston SA: Genetic immunization is a simple method for eliciting an immune response. Nature 1992 (356):152-154

52 Greenburg PD and Riddell SR: Tumor-specific T-cell immunity: ready for prime time? JNCI 1992 (84):1059-1061

53 Skerra A and Pluckthün A: Assembly of a functional immunoglobulin Fv fragment in *Escherichia coli*. Science 1988 (240): 1038-1041

54 Lemarchand P, Jaffe HA, Danel C, Cid MC, Kleinman HK, Stratford-Perricaudet LD, Perricaudet M, Pavirani A, Lecocq J-P and Crystal RG: Adenovirus-mediated transfer of a recombinant human a1-antitrypsin cDNA to human endothelial cells. Proc Natl Acad Sci USA. 1992 (89): 6482-6486

55 Felgner PL and Rhodes G: Gene Therapeutics. Nature 1991 (349):351-352

56 Wagner E, Zatlouski K, Cotten M, Kirlappos H, Mechtler K, Curiel DT and Birnsreil M: Coupling of adenovirus to transferrin-polylysine/DNA complexes greatly enhances receptor-mediated gene delivery and expression of transfected genes. Proc Natl Acad Sci USA 1992 (89):6099-6103

57 Leonetti J-P, Machy P, Degols G, Lebleu B and Leserman L: Antibody-targeted liposomes containing oligodeoxyribonucleotides complementary to viral RNA selectively inhibit viral replication. Proc Natl Acad Sci USA 1990 (87):2448-2451

58 Roux P, Jeanteur P and Piechaczyk M: A versatile and potentially general approach to the targeting of specific cell types by retroviruses: application to the infection of human cels by means of major histocompatibility complex class I and class II antigens by mouse ecotropic murine leukaemia virus derived viruses. Proc Natl Acad Sci USA 1989 (86):9079-9083

59 Trubetsky VS, Torchilin VP, Kennel SJ and Huang L: Use of N-terminal modified poly(l-lysine)-antibody conjugate as a carrier for targeted gene delivery in mouse lung endothelial cells. Bioconjugate Chem 1992 (3):323-327

60 Russell SJ, Hawkins RE, Winter G: Retroviral vectors displaying functional antibody fragments. Nucl Acids Res 1993 (21):1081-1086